RB 1843 402645 9001
Dun Laoghaire-Rathdown Libraries
GLENCULLEN LIBRARY
Inv/06 : K570 Price E21.90
Title: Diabetic cookbook
D0230005
BAINTE DEN STOC
WITHDRAWN FROM
DÚN LAOGHAIRE-RATHDOWN COUNTY
LIBRARY STOCK

THE DIABETIC COOKBOOK

100 QUICK AND EASY RECIPES

Good Housekeeping

THE DIABETIC COOKBOOK

100 QUICK AND EASY RECIPES

AZMINA GOVINDJI

COLLINS & BROWN

Current advice is that it is not harmful to include small amounts of sugar in a healthy diabetic diet. If you have not seen a dietitian recently, ask your GP to refer you so you get up to date guidance on sugar and other aspects of your diet.

First published in Great Britain in 2005 by Collins & Brown Limited
The Chrysalis Building
Bramley Road
London W10 6SP

Copyright © Collins & Brown Limited 2005
Text copyright and photographs copyright © The National Magazine Company Limited 2005

All rights reserved. No part of this publication may be reproduced, stored in a retrieval system, or transmitted in any form or by any means, electronic, mechanical, photocopying, recording or otherwise, without the prior written consent of the copyright holder.

The expression GOOD HOUSEKEEPING as used in the title of the book is the trademark of The National Magazine Company and The Hearst Corporation, registered in the United Kingdom and USA, and other principle countries of the world, and is the absolute property of The National Magazine Company and The Hearst Corporation. The use of this trademark other than with the express permission of The National Magazine Company or The Hearst Corporation is strictly prohibited.

The Good Housekeeping website address is www.goodhousekeeping.co.uk

2 3 4 5 6 7 8 9
British Library Cataloguing-in-Publication Data:
A catalogue record for this book is available from the British Library.

ISBN 1-84340-264-5

Project Editor: Nicola Hodgson
Designer: Lotte Oldfield
Typesetter: Ben Cracknell
Proofreader: Fiona Corbridge
Nutritional analysis: Jenny McGlyne
Indexer: Michèle Clark

Reproduction by Anorax Ltd
Printed and bound by CT Printing, China

This book was typeset using Abadi

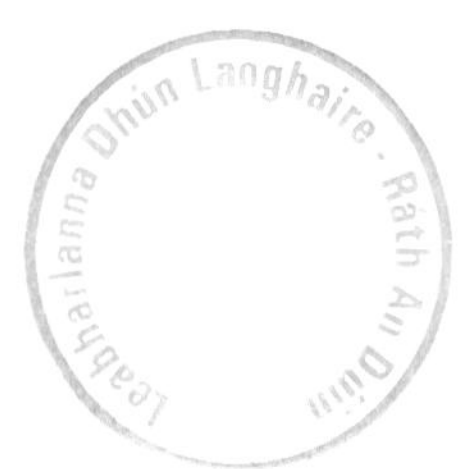

CONTENTS

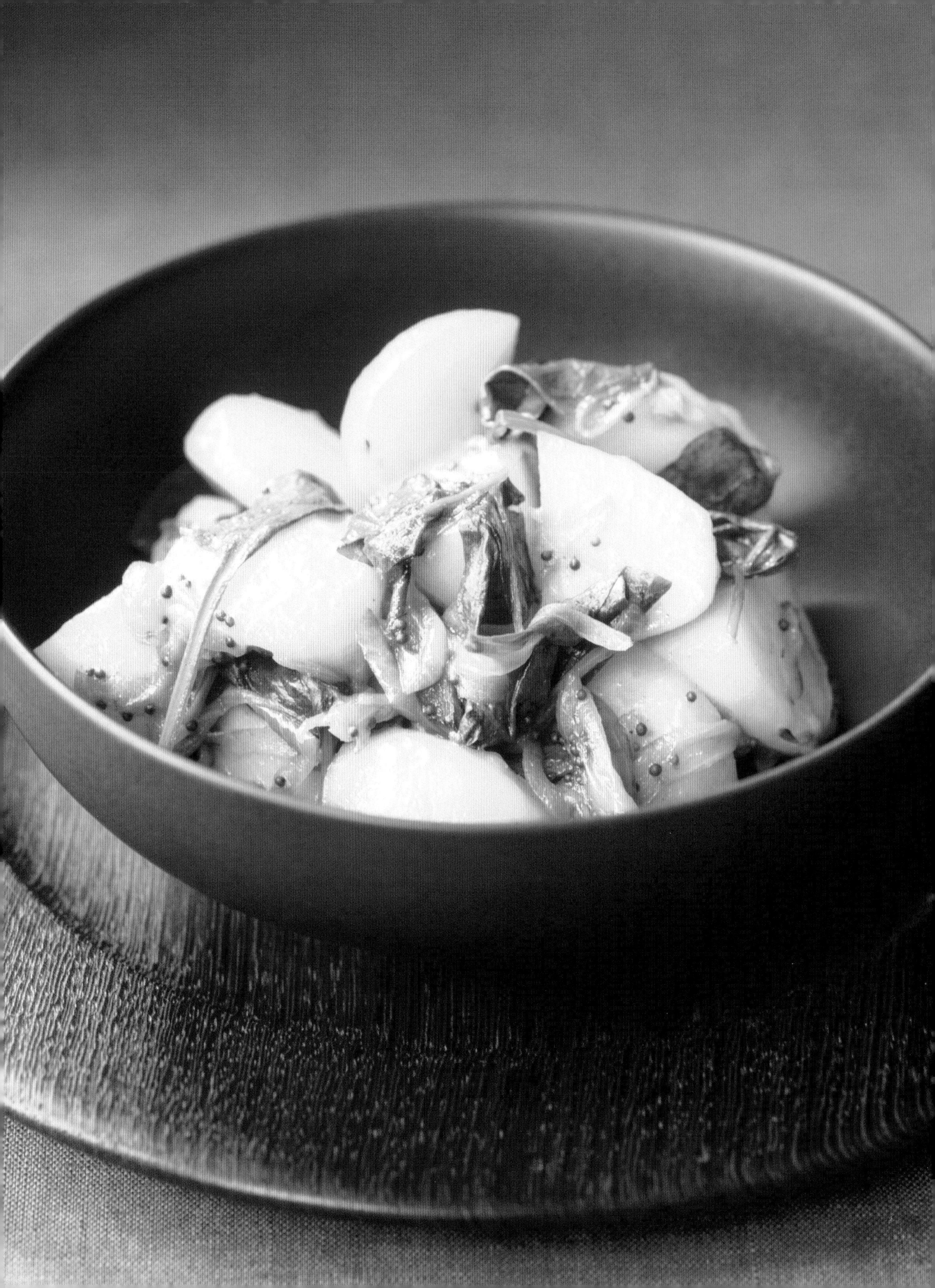

FOREWORD

A good diet is more important to someone with diabetes than it is to even the most ardent gastronome. Far beyond offering mere pleasure to the taste buds, it forms the cornerstone of successful blood glucose control and offers a lifetime free from the complications of diabetes, which can be so devastating.

Of course, eating healthily requires conscious effort, but the rewards can be very far-reaching. Published in 1998, the UKPDS (United Kingdom Prospective Diabetes Study) quantified the benefits of good control of blood glucose levels and blood pressure, showing that in type 2 diabetes the risk of heart disease could be reduced by 56 per cent, stroke by 44 per cent, and kidney disease by up to 33 per cent. Medication and exercise play a vital role too, but understanding how to eat well is paramount.

Thankfully, today, our improved understanding of nutrition and the wonderfully cosmopolitan array of foods available to shoppers mean that the diabetic diet is not the drab, uninspiring affair of yesterday. The recipes included here successfully marry the benefits of healthy eating with the sumptuous delights of tasty, but easily prepared, meals. This book certainly proves that being diagnosed with diabetes no longer spells the end of enjoyable eating.

At the Diabetes Research & Wellness Foundation, we are acutely aware of the need to stress the importance of healthy eating and daily exercise to people with diabetes. Worryingly, the current figure of 1.8 million people in the United Kingdom diagnosed with diabetes is expected to increase to 3 million by the end of the decade, so it is vital that the message gets across loud and clear. Our campaigns, educational events and literature are aimed at improving understanding of diabetes, as well as reaching and informing those at risk of developing this potentially life-threatening condition.

Being diagnosed with diabetes presents an enormous challenge but with the right help and necessary support, life can still be lived to the full. Anyone seeking advice, reassurance or information is encouraged to contact us at the Diabetes Research & Wellness Foundation. We also welcome new members who want to become part of a network of people with diabetes, their families and friends.

Please visit our website at www.drwf.org.uk for more information or write to us at: 101–102, Northney Marina, Hayling Is. Hampshire. PO11 0NH. Tel: 023 9263 7808.

James A.S. Rogers LL.B.
Executive Director
Diabetes Research & Wellness Foundation

INTRODUCTION

Diabetes is a life-long condition – not a life sentence. It is simply something that needs looking after, and if you take a few easy steps to ensure your health is a priority for you, you can still enjoy a full life. The first step is understanding what diabetes is, then what it means to you, personally. If you treat your health and diabetes as a priority today by following a few simple guidelines, you will have an abundance of healthy tomorrows – it's up to you.

Make you a priority

You will only be able to look after those special people around you if you first look after yourself. Allow yourself to take time to explore your needs, to understand your condition, or indeed, understand the diabetes of someone close to you, if you are a carer. The more you know about how you can keep your diabetes in check, the more you will be able to enjoy everything that life has to offer – as well as the challenges it throws at you.

Picking up this book is one way you have chosen to acknowledge the importance of healthy changes in your life. As you take on the practical tips given in this introduction, and indulge in the mouthwatering recipes, you will see the changes come to life, on your plate; on your waistline and in your overall sense of well being. Worth a bit of your time? Then let's begin ...

What is diabetes?

When you have diabetes, the amount of glucose (sugar) in your blood is too high because your body cannot use it properly. Glucose comes mainly from the digestion of starchy foods such as pasta, rice and potatoes, and sweet foods such as sugary drinks and cakes. The glucose triggers the release of a hormone called insulin, which is needed for the body to use the glucose as fuel or energy.

If there is not enough insulin, or if the insulin you have is not working efficiently enough, glucose can build up in your blood. This is called hyperglycaemia and you can be tested for this by having a Glucose Tolerance Test (GTT) at the local hospital. A positive result generally leads to the diagnosis of diabetes. If you have the following symptoms, it is advisable to ask your GP to test your urine (you can also do this at home with urine testing strips from the pharmacy). If glucose is found in your urine, you will be asked to have a GTT to confirm whether you have diabetes. Symptoms of diabetes include thirst and a dry mouth, passing large amounts of urine (especially at night), loss of weight, tiredness, genital itchiness and blurring of vision.

If diabetes is not addressed, you are at risk of long-term health complications. These include heart disease, nerve damage (so you might get loss of sensation in your toes and fingers), kidney disease, vision impairment (even blindness) and other problems. If you are overweight, you are particularly at risk of type 2 diabetes, the most common type. So, the recipes in this book are all calorie-counted and low in fat, helping you to make appropriate choices in terms of your weight, heart health and diabetes. They are also suitable and healthy for the whole family, whether you have diabetes or not. If you have diabetes, you already have an increased risk of developing heart disease, so watching what you eat is even more important. This cookbook could make a big difference to your life – if you choose to take the advice on board.

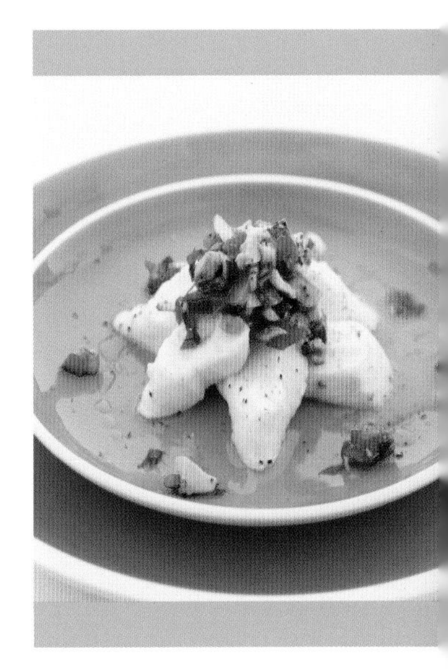

Types of diabetes

There are two main types of diabetes:

Type 1 diabetes *(or insulin-dependent diabetes)* occurs when the body has a severe lack of insulin. It is treated by insulin injections and a healthy way of eating, based on regular meals and snacks. It usually occurs in people under 40 years of age. There are many different types of insulin, which affect the body in different ways, and your diabetes specialists will work with you to find the treatment that's best for you.

Type 2 diabetes *(or non-insulin-dependent diabetes)* is the most common type and about 75 per cent of people with diabetes are in this category. The body can still make some insulin, but this is not enough for its needs. People with type 2 diabetes are usually overweight and are advised to reduce weight by eating a range of healthy foods; and some people may need tablets in addition. It usually affects people over about 40 years of age, but with rising rates of obesity, more and more type 2 diabetes is being diagnosed at a younger age, even in children, and especially in overweight, inactive children.

Some people require insulin to treat their diabetes but are not truly insulin-dependent. They may be treated by tablets and insulin injections within an overall balanced eating plan.

There is no cure for diabetes, and there is no such thing as mild diabetes. However, with the appropriate treatment and a healthy attitude, you can enjoy a full and active life. Keeping diabetes in check is based on keeping your blood glucose levels within an optimum range. The food you eat has a direct effect on your blood glucose – which is good news. It's good because you are in control of what you eat – you have the power to do something significant about your diabetes.

The food connection

What you eat, and how often you eat makes your blood glucose levels fluctuate, and the aim is therefore to achieve slow, steady rises and falls in blood glucose throughout the day, a bit like slow waves going up and down. It makes sense – if you eat, your blood glucose goes up and different foods will make it go up more or less slowly. If you choose foods that make it go up slowly, that is better for your diabetes. If you eat regularly, you are more likely to achieve the slow, steady waves than if you miss meals or indulge in heavy meals and then starve yourself because you feel guilty. Work with your body, listen to it, and it will reward you.

There is no such thing as a special diabetic diet, and a range of healthy foods such as the dishes in this book can be beneficial whether you have diabetes or not. As each person varies in their dietary requirements, it is recommended that people diagnosed with diabetes visit a registered dietitian for tailored dietary advice.

People with diabetes used to be advised to restrict the use of sugar and sugary foods. However, you do not need to avoid sugar completely. Research shows that when you eat sugar as part of a balanced, healthy diet it will not have a harmful effect on blood glucose control. So, do include some sugar if you like, especially if you are not overweight, but be sure to take it in the context of a healthy diet. The key is to get the balance right. Having a dessert on occasions after a meal should not cause blood sugar to rise too quickly. If you are overweight, you need to look at the calorie content of the recipes and choose those that are lower in calories.

DIETARY GUIDELINES FOR DIABETES

- Eat regular meals and snacks and choose lower glycaemic starchy foods (see tables opposite) like grainy bread, pasta, oats, beans, lentils, fruit and vegetables.
- Watch your intake of fried and fatty foods such as butter, full-fat cheese, fatty meats, crisps and pastries. Choose lower fat cooking methods (see page 21).
- Eat five portions of fruit and vegetables a day (see Eating to your Heart's Content, page 13).
- Replace high-sugar foods (such as tinned fruit in syrup; sugared drinks) with low-sugar foods (such as tinned fruit in natural juice; sugar-free drinks).
- Eat a portion of oily fish once a week. Research suggests that this can significantly reduce the incidence of heart disease, and it even benefits those people who have already suffered a heart attack. Try Japanese-style Salmon or Lemon Tuna (pages 85 and 90).
- Keep an eye on how much salt you use. A high salt intake is linked with high blood pressure.
- Limit the amount of alcohol you drink (see page 16).

The Glycaemic Index (GI)

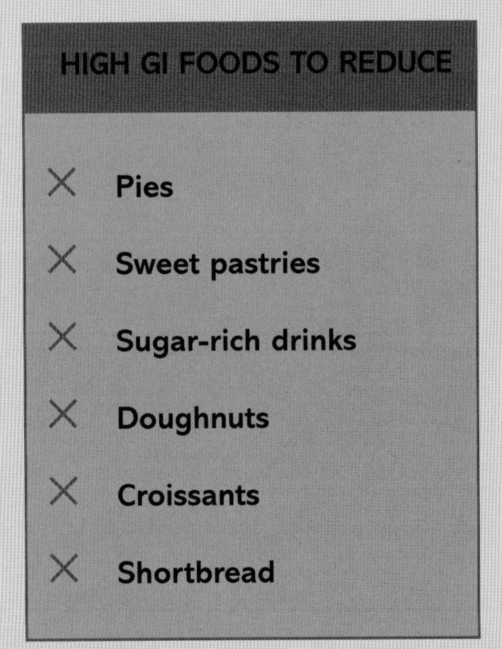

HEALTHY LOW GI FOODS

- ✓ **Pasta** (choose tomato-based sauces)
- ✓ **Grainy breads** (such as soya and linseed, granary)
- ✓ **Bran-based** (not flaked) **breakfast cereals**
- ✓ **Porridge** and reduced sugar muesli
- ✓ **Sweet potatoes** and new boiled potatoes in skins
- ✓ **Nuts** (limit to a small handful a day)
- ✓ **Fruits**
- ✓ **Vegetables** (raw or lightly cooked)
- ✓ **Salad** (choose low-fat dressings)
- ✓ **Basmati rice**

The GI is a ranking of foods, which tells us how they affect blood glucose levels. The faster a food is broken down during digestion, the quicker blood glucose rises. Since one of the main aims of treatment of diabetes is to keep blood glucose levels steady throughout the day, foods that cause sharp rises in blood glucose are best kept to a minimum (unless needed for special circumstances, such as illness, hypoglycaemia or exercise). Foods that cause a rapid rise in blood glucose have a high GI, so the key is to choose more foods with a low GI regularly.

In general, wholegrains (for example, granary bread, porridge and muesli), fruit, vegetables, nuts, beans and lentils have a low to medium GI and it makes sense to base meals and snacks on these foods. It doesn't mean this is all you should eat. Variety is vitality – vary your foods to get a wide range of nutrients and you are more likely to get those vital vitamins and minerals needed for good health. Although low GI foods, like those mentioned above, tend to be vegetarian, this doesn't mean that meat is not appropriate for diabetes. In fact, lean red meat is an excellent source of iron. Because meat doesn't have any carbohydrate, it will not raise your blood glucose levels. But it is still best to limit the amount you eat, as too much protein may be potentially damaging to your kidneys. Since people with diabetes are already at an increased risk of developing kidney disease, low-carb high-protein diets are not recommended.

Instead, choose to follow a plan that encourages foods with a low GI within the context of overall healthy balanced eating (see page 138, Further Support and Information). The main thing to remember is that a low-GI food is digested slowly and causes a slow and steady rise (and fall) in blood glucose. Slow digestion can help to make you feel full for longer and delay hunger pangs. In this way, it is easier for you to eat well, lose weight if you need to, and keep an eye on your diabetes. You don't have to cut out all high GI foods. It is better to think about the overall balance of your meals, as we usually eat foods in combination (see the diagram on page 20). The good thing is you can lower the overall GI of a meal by including more low GI foods such as vegetables or salads.

Here are some basic guidelines:

1. Have one low-GI food at each meal or snack (also see Shopping and cooking for diabetes, page 23).

2. Buy grainy breads made with whole seeds, barley and oats instead of white, wholemeal or brown bread. (Since the grains have been processed in wholemeal bread, it is digested more quickly than granary, where the grains are still whole.)

3. Choose breakfast cereals based on wholegrains such as porridge oats and muesli.

4. Wheat-based pasta, sweet potatoes and basmati rice are great low-GI foods – enjoy them regularly and use the low-fat cooking methods as shown in the recipes in this book.

5. Dairy foods tend to be low GI and are high in calcium – enjoy skimmed or semi-skimmed milk and low-fat yogurt two to three times a day. If going for cheese, have 25g (1oz) of ordinary cheese or 50g (2oz) of reduced-fat cheese as a serving. Grating stronger cheeses helps you to use less.

6. Eat more beans, lentils and peas. Throw them into stews, casseroles, or simply spice them up with lemon and chilli for a snack. Recipes such as Chilli Con Carne (page 60) and Turkey, Pepper and Haricot Casserole (page 79) are perfect examples.

7. Go for whole fruits rather than fruit juices. A juice will be digested and absorbed quickly, so your blood glucose will rise more rapidly, which is undesirable. Low-GI fruits include apples, dried apricots, cherries, grapefruit, grapes, orange, peaches, pears, plums and firm bananas.

8. Eat fruit and vegetables raw, or just cooked, rather than overcooked, and eat them whole rather than mashed and puréed.

9. Fill up on fibre by choosing foods such as beans, lentils, fruit, vegetables and fibre-rich breakfast cereals. Fibre helps slow the digestion and absorption of starchy foods and also can give you a feeling of fullness.

10. Most vegetables and fruits have a low GI rating, and are low in calories and fat – they are your best friends.

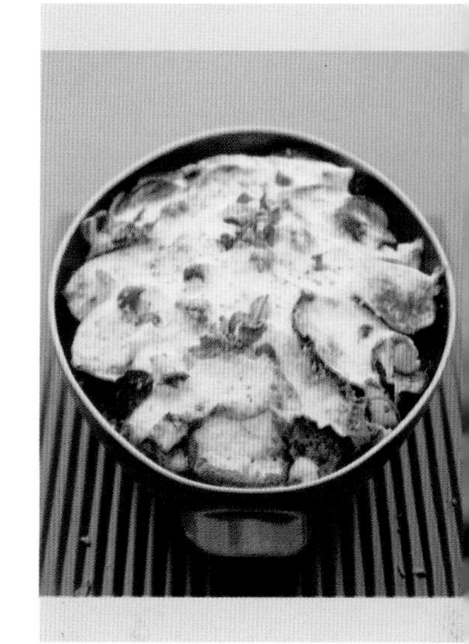

Eating to your heart's content

Heart disease is more common in people with diabetes. Over the years, especially if you eat foods that are rich in saturated fat and have an inactive lifestyle, fats in the blood can get deposited on the walls of the arteries around the heart. As the fats harden, they fur up the vessel (a process called atherosclerosis). If these deposits get damaged, they trigger the formation of a blood clot (thrombosis), which blocks the already narrowed vessel. A narrow artery can completely cut off the blood and oxygen supply to the heart and this kills part of the heart muscle, causing a heart attack.

People with type 2 diabetes often share a collection of medical conditions which encourage this process. They include:

- High blood pressure
- Abnormal blood fats including raised 'bad' (LDL) cholesterol and low 'good' cholesterol (HDL)
- 'Sticky blood' with an increased tendency to form clots
- High levels of an amino acid called homocysteine in the blood

The good news is that these conditions can all be improved by a healthy lifestyle – which includes stopping smoking and taking regular physical activity (see page 22). Losing excess weight and keeping it off are also very effective (see page 17).

However, there's more good news – eating for a healthy heart isn't all about cutting back on tasty foods. Let's take a look at the many enjoyable foods that are positively good for the heart – you may be in for a few surprises!

Fat facts

Unsaturated fats from vegetable oils and fish help lower blood cholesterol and reduce the risk of blood clots. It's a good idea to replace fats for cooking and spreading with a product based on these oils. Monounsaturated fats as found in rapeseed and olive oil are particularly good and are probably the key reason why people in Mediterranean countries have relatively lower rates of heart disease.

However, eating a lot of fat, especially saturated (animal) fat raises blood cholesterol, which can get deposited on artery walls. Cutting down on fatty meats and meat products, full-fat dairy foods, fried foods, butter and pastries, cakes and biscuits will help.

Watch out too for 'trans' fats, which are unsaturated fats that have been hydrogenated (a type of processing) to make them harder. These have also been shown to raise cholesterol and promote blood clots and weight for weight, they are worse for the heart than saturates. They can be found in a variety of foods, from margarines and spreads, to baked foods to takeaways.

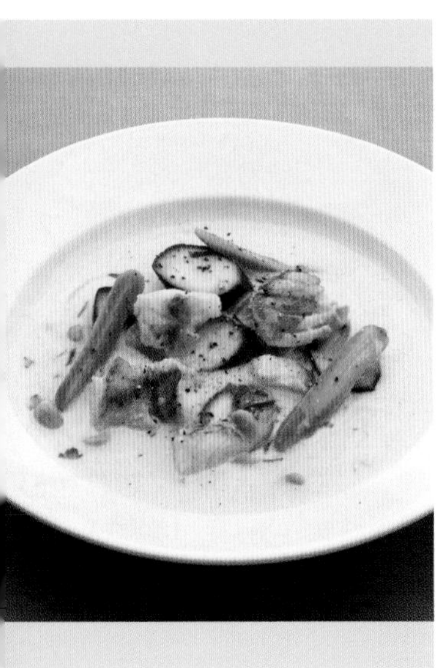

Take five!

Fruit and vegetables contain a whole cocktail of beneficial nutrients which protect the heart. These include vitamins such as beta-carotene, vitamin C and folic acid, which help prevent narrowing of the arteries. They're also a rich source of potassium – known for its beneficial effects on lowering blood pressure. Studies have clearly shown that high dietary intakes of both fruit and vegetables are related to a lower risk of heart disease. Unfortunately, you don't get the same benefit from popping a vitamin pill. Try to eat a variety of types and colours of fruit and vegetables, aiming for a minimum of five portions a day. Current UK intakes are well below this, at only two to three portions a day. Fresh, frozen, tinned and dried types can contribute to this total and all are suitable for people with diabetes.

Remember that pulses such as beans and lentils count only once a day as they contain fewer of the heart-protecting nutrients than other fruits and vegetables. Fruit juice will be more rapidly absorbed, even if it is unsweetened, as most of the valuable soluble fibre will have been removed. Potatoes are considered to be a starchy food and don't count as one of your five a day target.

Fishy tips

The recommended intake is two servings of fish per week (one of which should be oily). Oily fish contain a type of unsaturated fat known as omega 3. This has a multitude of magical effects on the heart including reducing stickiness of the blood, blood pressure and irregular heart rhythms. Studies have shown that regularly eating oily fish dramatically reduces the incidence of heart attacks, especially in people who have already had one. Examples of oily fish include salmon, herrings, sardines, pilchards, mackerel, trout and fresh tuna. Vegetarian sources of omega 3 oils include soy, linseed (flaxseed), walnuts and rapeseed oil.

Halt the salt

Too much salt can be bad for the heart. It has been shown to provoke an increase in blood pressure, particularly as you get older. You need a small amount of salt for your body to function normally, but most of us eat far too much – around 9–12g (1½ to 2 tsp) a day. It is recommended that you take no more than 6g (about 1 tsp) per day.

Around three-quarters of our salt intake comes from manufactured foods, and weight for weight many of these are saltier than sea water. Checking the label can help you to choose low-salt products.

In practice, reducing salt means less reliance on processed foods, ready meals, salty snacks and takeaways, and more use of fresh ingredients. Sounds like common sense – and if you choose fewer processed foods, you are more likely to be taking in carbs with a lower GI rating (see page 11). Many of the recipes in this book have been specifically created to help you keep your salt addition to a minimum. Herbs, spices and other flavours have been used to help provide an interesting array of tastes and avoid excessive use of added salt.

Gradually reducing salt at the table and in cooking can help too – studies show taste buds quickly adapt. Meanwhile, you can use other herbs, spices, garlic, pepper and lime juice as flavours. Neither iodized and sea salt are better for your blood pressure, but salt substitutes based on potassium chloride can be useful for some people. They contain 30–70 per cent less but are not suitable for people who have kidney problems.

Wholegrain truths

Wholegrain cereals and bread contain a range of heart-friendly nutrients. Many big surveys have shown that eating wholegrain foods protects against heart disease. Recommendations are to aim for two to three helpings per day but in the UK only one in five of us achieves this. Many of the foods in this group also have a low glycaemic index or GI (see pages 11–12) making them good choices for people with diabetes.

Dairy dividends

Low-fat dairy foods are a rich source of calcium which, together with vitamin D, helps keep bones strong. Recent studies have shown that calcium also plays a role in helping to lower blood pressure. Current advice is to aim for three servings a day of lower-fat varieties of milk, cheese or yogurt. (A serving is a glass of milk, a carton of yogurt or a matchbox-sized piece of cheese.)

Calcium-enriched soya milks, cheeses, yogurts and soya bean curd (tofu) are a good alternative to dairy products. Eating soya foods two to three times a day brings the added bonus of helping to lower cholesterol levels.

Here's to your good health

Having a drink can be one of life's great pleasures, but it's all about getting the balance right. Alcoholic drinks are measured in units. A unit is a small glass of wine, a standard measure of spirits, or half a pint of normal-strength beer. Light drinking (less than 1–2 units of alcohol per day) seems to offer some protection against heart disease by increasing 'good' cholesterol and reducing the risk of blood clots. Wine, spirits and even beer work, but it is men over 40 and post-menopausal women who benefit most. Unfortunately more isn't better and levels greater than 2–3 units a day for women and 3–4 units per day for men increase health risk from high blood pressure, liver damage and even cancer. Observe the safe drinking limit for everyone: 21–28 units a week for men (or 3–4 units a day) and 14–21 units a week for women (or 2–3 units a day). These are the maximum recommended amounts – it's better to drink less.

KNOW YOUR UNITS

1 unit of alcohol = ½ pint beer or lager = 1 pub measure of sherry, aperitif or liqueur = 1 standard glass or wine = 1 pub measure of spirits, such as vodka or gin.

Safe drinking

Alcohol can cause hypoglycaemia (a 'hypo', or low blood glucose) if you are taking insulin or certain tablets for your diabetes. Drinks that have a high alcohol content, such as spirits, are more likely to cause a hypo. Here are a few guidelines to help prevent this happening:

- Avoid drinking on an empty stomach. Always have something to eat (such as a handful of peanuts) with a drink and especially after going out drinking (for example, oat biscuits and milk, or a sandwich). This is because the hypoglycaemic effect of alcohol can last for several hours.
- Choose low-alcohol drinks in preference to those that are higher in alcohol.
- Avoid special diabetic or low-carbohydrate beers or lagers, as these tend to be higher in alcohol.
- If you enjoy spirits, try to use sugar-free or slimline mixers.
- If you count the amount of carbohydrate you eat, don't include the carbohydrate from alcoholic drinks.
- Drink less alcohol if you are trying to lose weight (limit yourself to about 1 unit a day).

Nutritious nuts

You may think nuts are out of bounds, as they are simply too fattening. However, they contain mainly the beneficial kind of monounsaturated fat found in olive oil. In addition, they're packed full of vitamins, minerals and fibre. Recent studies suggest that eating small amounts (about a handful) of nuts such as peanuts or almonds 4–5 times a week as a snack or alternative protein food can help reduce heart disease. They also have a low GI and 25g (1oz) a day, as part of a healthy diet, can help you lose weight. Unsalted are best since, as we've seen above, most of us already get far too much salt as it is.

What about cholesterol in foods?

Foods such as eggs and shellfish contain dietary cholesterol. However, in most people this has very little effect compared with the cholesterol that is made by your liver in response to a high animal fat diet. Unless advised otherwise by your diabetes team, eating these foods in sensible amounts as part of a healthy diet should not increase your risk of heart disease.

Plant sterols

'Functional foods' claim to give a health benefit over and above the basic nutrient content, usually from an added ingredient. The plant *stanol* or *sterol esters* are commonly promoted for heart disease and are added to foods such as margarine, yogurt, yogurt drink and soft cheese spread. The claims are based on good evidence showing useful reductions in blood cholesterol levels as part of a healthy diet. However, you do need to take the recommended dose to get a benefit and it is really important to continue to eat enough fruit and vegetables, as plant sterols can reduce the absorption of beta-carotene.

Weight matters!

You now know that the type of food you eat affects both short-term blood sugar control and the long-term risk of complications from diabetes, such as heart disease. However the quantity of food consumed, especially the amount of energy it contains (measured as calories or kcals), also matters significantly.

Most people with type 2 diabetes are overweight. Indeed, being overweight might have been the trigger to their development of diabetes in the first place. The chart overleaf will help you to tell if you are one of these people. Carrying excess weight, especially around the middle, will reduce your sensitivity to insulin and make managing diabetes more difficult. Losing weight can really help. It will also help reduce your risk of heart disease, arthritis, gallstones, gout and several types of cancer.

How to tell if you are overweight:

1. Get your weight right

The chart on page 18 will help you to find out just how much weight you need to lose to be within a healthy range. Plot your weight on the left-hand axis (without clothes). Do the same with the horizontal axis for your height (without shoes). Make a straight line from each mark and note where the two lines meet. This will show you what your body mass index is – your target weight will be in the 'healthy weight range'. If you are overweight, start by aiming for the higher end of this range for now. Once you have maintained your new weight for a few months, you can aim for a lower weight closer to the middle of this range.

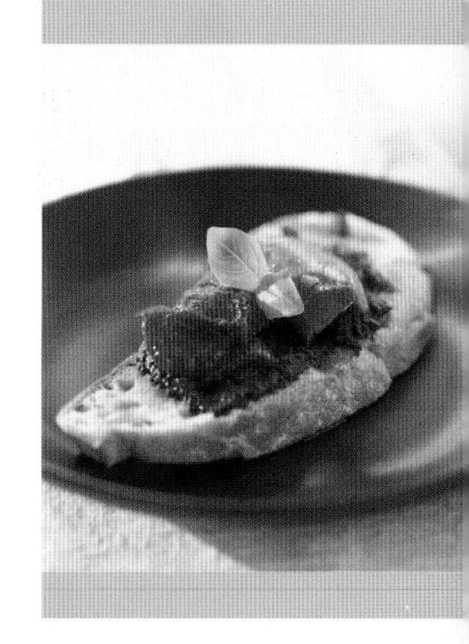

2. Measure your waist

If your waist is bigger than your hips (you are an 'apple' shape), you are more likely to suffer long- term conditions such as heart disease than if your waist is smaller than your hips ('pear' shaped). This is so significant that the British Dietetic Association Food First Campaign for 2002–2004, called Weight Wise, extensively published the following guidelines:

At-risk waist measurement for European men	94cm (37in)
At-risk waist measurement for European and South Asian women	80cm (32in)
At-risk waist measurement for South Asian men	90cm (36in)

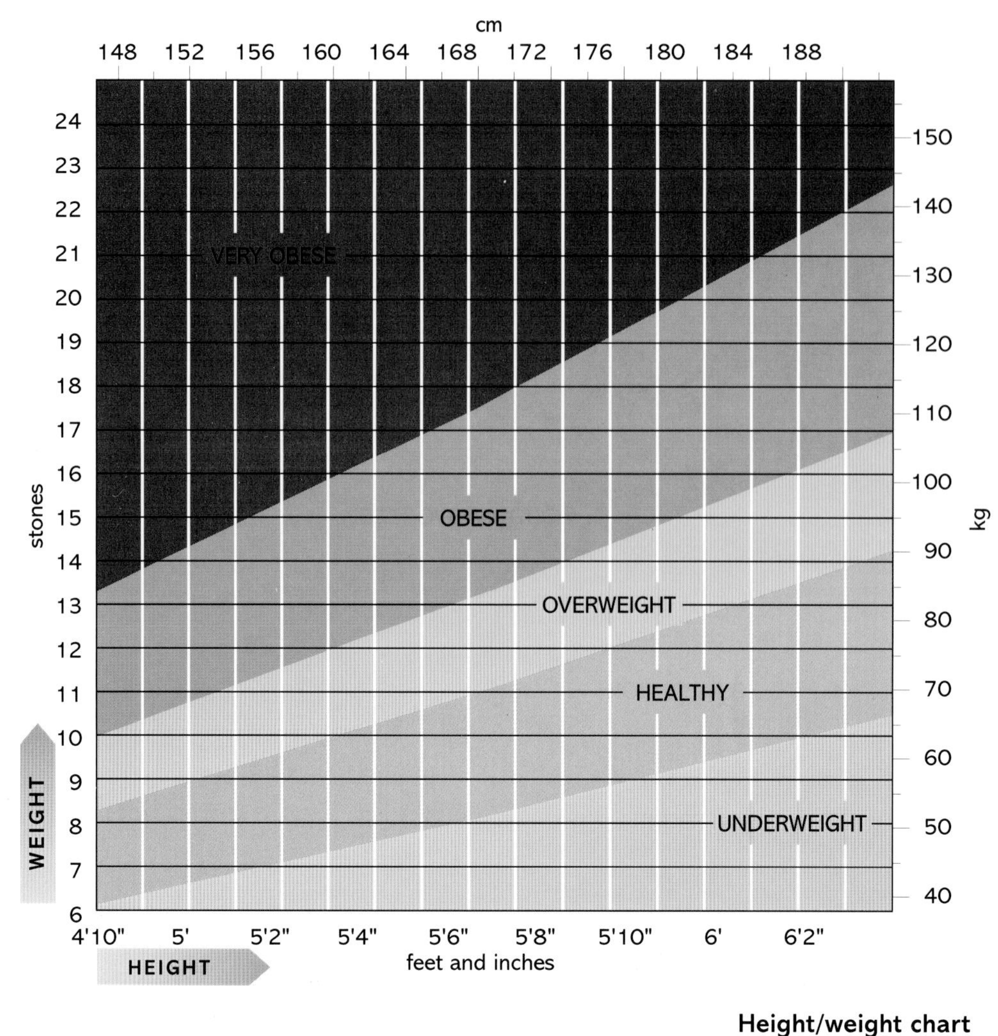

Height/weight chart

How can I successfully lose weight?

Recent surveys have shown that most of us manage to lose some weight when we start a new diet. Unfortunately most of us put it all back on when we stop!

The UK diet industry is the second largest in Europe. Last year, 34 million Britons tried to lose weight, with an average spend of £300 per slimmer, on diet products. Most of us are unclear about what does and doesn't work, and mixed messages are given by the media and sometimes even by well-meaning health writers. In this section we look at the approaches we know really do help with weight loss.

Step 1: Set yourself a target you can reach

When asked, most dieters generally state their goal as reaching their 'ideal weight'. For some people that can be quite a distant land and may not be very realistic. Few dieters are aware that losing just 10 per cent of their body weight will have real health benefits. For example, an 83kg (13 stone) adult losing 8.3kg (1 stone 4lbs) will not only feel and look better but will see noticeable improvements in blood sugar control, blood fats and blood pressure. The first step on the road to successful weight loss is to set yourself a target you can achieve. You can always review it at a later date if you feel you can lose more.

Step 2: Be realistic about weekly weight loss rates

Most people want to lose weight fast. Bookshops are heaving with titles claiming to show how you can do just that. However, studies have shown that rapid weight loss causes you to lose proportionally more muscle tissue and increases the likelihood that you'll regain the weight. The ideal rate seems to be between 0.5–1kg (1–2lb) a week. This can be achieved by cutting your food intake by just 500 kcal per day and is both safe and manageable. Remember, the weight did not go on overnight so it's not going to come off safely that way either! So, if you are going for a slimming diet, try one that offers you slow, sustainable weight loss such as a balanced low-GI (glycaemic index) plan (visit www.giplan.com). You are likely to feel less hungry following such a plan, which means you will be able to keep to it for longer. Ideally, go for a weight loss plan that means simple changes to your overall lifestyle – one that you can keep to in the long term.

Step 3: Steer clear of fad diets

Don't be tempted by the outrageous claims of miracle diets. One of main reasons dieters give up and regain weight is that they're fed up following difficult and boring diets. To date there are no magic bullets for weight loss. As a guide, avoid any diet that tells you to cut out whole food groups or encourages you to eat lots of one particular food. Culprits include the cabbage soup and grapefruit diets, food combining, detox and blood group diets, and variants of the low-carbohydrate diet. From experience, if a diet plan sounds too good to be true then it probably is!

Traditional low-carbohydrate diets, encourage unlimited amounts of red meat, fish, cheese and fatty foods such as cream and butter. Bread, potatoes, pasta and rice, as well as many fruit and vegetables are usually restricted. Followers of the diet are advised to take supplements to make up for any nutrients they are missing out on. These diets are the least suitable for people with diabetes, especially those on medication. They provide insufficient carbohydrate and are very likely to be high in protein, which could be potentially damaging to the kidneys. The most extreme phases of the diet fly in the face of widely accepted healthy-eating guidelines which we know protect against chronic health problems such as heart disease and cancer.

Dieters sometimes like the novelty of a fad diet and lose weight well at first. However, given time many report that the diets become tedious and impractical, not to mention costly. A balanced approach, which incorporates all the food groups within the context of an overall low-GI diet is far more appropriate for diabetes. See page 138 for further information on low-GI diets.

Step 4: Choose some small but lasting changes you can make to your diet

Most of us eat far too much fat and sugar. As a result our diets are very high in energy or calories. Scientists have suggested that today's diet, containing lots of fast foods and takeaways, is over twice as high in calories as that of our ancestors. There are many ways to make small changes to reduce this (see the table on page 21). Why not select some that you think you could easily incorporate and move on to others with time?

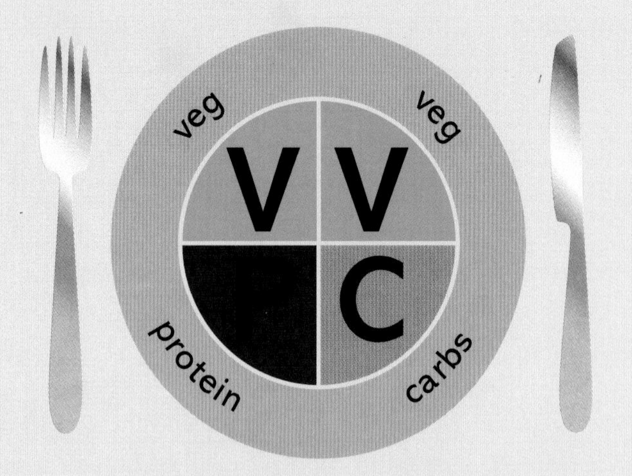

Imagining your plate split into these sections will help you get the balance of foods right.

Step 5: Get the balance right

Taking on all the advice and being aware of balance in every meal can be difficult. A great tip for helping you to choose wisely and automatically have a more balanced, slimming yet filling meal, is to imagine your plate is split into four quarters. Now, fill two of these quarters with veg (such as crunchy broccoli and carrots), one with low-GI carbs (such as pasta), and one with protein (such as chargrilled meat or fish). Look at the picture, left, and take it with you in your mind whenever you sit down to a meal. To help you, just remember the letters V (veggie), V (veggie), P (protein), C (carbs) or V V P C – simple!

Step 6: Watch those portion sizes

Over the last few years, portion sizes of many of our favourite foods have been gradually creeping up without us noticing. This includes not only snack foods such as chocolate bars, crisps and sandwiches, but also ready meals, drinks, takeaways and restaurant meals. An average portion of chips has gone up from around 300 kcals to over 500 kcals, a bag of crisps from 140 kcals to as much as 270 kcals and a glass of wine in the pub from around 95kcals to over 180 kcals. One well-known chain of family restaurants now actually serves a main course containing over 2000 kcalories!

Interestingly, studies on supersized sandwiches showed that consumers were no more satisfied by the larger portions and did not compensate by eating less later on in the day. If you eat these foods, make sure you look at the label and where possible go for the smaller sizes. If not, you risk taking in a lot more than you intended! Fill up on extra vegetables, salad or fruit and feel virtuous at the end of the day rather than guilty.

Step 7: Think about how and why you eat

Keeping a food and mood diary for a few days can give you a great insight into your behaviour around eating which has led to weight gain in the first place. It can show you the reasons other than hunger for eating (such as boredom or stress), and enable you to think of ways of dealing with these.

Make sure you don't go without foods for long periods at a time – you'll end up starving and eat more than you intended. Try to have breakfast each day: it could actually help you take in fewer calories.

Slowing down the speed at which you eat will give yourself time to feel full on less. Make sure you sit down to eat rather than grazing on the move or munching at your computer. Studies have shown clearly that dieters who take on board behavioural changes lose significantly more weight than those who don't.

USUAL FOOD	HEALTHIER OPTION
French fries or mashed potato	New potatoes boiled in their skins.
Fatty meat	Select lean cuts of meat with visible fat removed, poultry without the skin, fish. Try to cook meat without adding fat by grilling, roasting and braising. Avoid using the juices from roast meat for gravy.
Flaky pastry	Filo pastry with skimmed milk between layers. Use occasionally.
Sugar-coated breakfast cereal	Muesli, porridge, high-fibre cereals.
Mayonnaise	Reduced-calorie mayonnaise or fat-free dressings.
Sugared fizzy drink	Unsweetened fruit juice, diet drink or water.
Rich iced cake, doughnut, cream-filled and chocolate biscuits	Fruit loaf, plain biscuits, oatcakes.
Rich desserts	Low-fat fruit yogurt, regular or reduced-calorie ice cream, fresh fruit, canned fruit in natural juice, sugar-free jelly, sugar-free, low fat instant desserts, 'light' or low-fat versions of tinned milk puddings and custard.
Full-fat dairy products, such as full-fat milk/cheese, butter	Reduced-fat dairy foods, such as semi-skimmed milk, half-fat cheese, reduced or low-fat spread.
Cooking oil for frying	Spray oil for greasing and stir- frying.
Sugar	Artificial sweeteners.

Try these tips:

- Eat on a smaller plate to make your meals look bigger.
- Avoid night-time snacking and TV dinners. Eat at a table and be conscious of what you're eating.
- Distract yourself at times when you feel like overindulging. Perhaps go for a stroll, take a bath or read a magazine.
- Never shop when you're hungry or you might go for those quick-fix snacks, and regret it later.
- Make a list of all the benefits of reaching your goal. This can be very motivating, so keep it handy.
- Encourage your family and friends to join in with your exercise regime. It's much more fun to go cycling, swimming or play sport with other people.

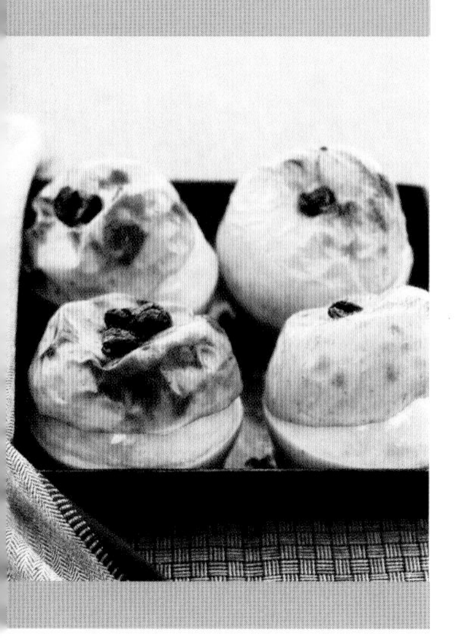

Step 8: Seek some support

Research has shown that most successful dieters have good support. It doesn't matter whether it's a friend, a partner or even an internet site. See Further Support and Information (page 138) for reputable internet sites and publications. Several big diet trials have shown that group approaches like slimming clubs can be both popular and successful. Long gone are the embarrassing group weigh-ins. The programmes are generally based on sound scientific principles usually using everyday foods and are easy to follow and understand.

Step 9: Be more active more often

Increasing your activity level while you're trying to lose weight will increase the amount of weight you lose and the proportion of fat lost. Most importantly, it will also help you to keep the weight off. There are many other health benefits from regular activity for someone with diabetes.

Physical activity helps your body to release endorphins, (natural painkillers), which can in turn help you combat stress and feel energized. It can also help you to achieve the body shape you want, and more importantly it has a host of health benefits. You don't need to jog ten times round the park or go to the gym every day in order to stay fit. Try to incorporate simple activities into your daily lifestyle and gradually try to work up to 30 minutes activity five times a week. It's fine to have three ten-minute bursts of activity; you don't need to be exercising for thirty minutes at a time.

- Walk to the letter box, take the dog out more often, take the kids for a brisk walk or simply park the car a bit further away from your destination. Try to walk at a pace that leaves you slightly out of breath.
- Use the stairs instead of the lift, or run up and down the stairs at home a few times a day.
- Try skipping or jogging on the spot whilst watching your favourite TV programme.
- Take up a sport that you enjoy and which fits into your routine. Swimming or line dancing classes with a friend can be a fun way of working out.

- Remember that activity can be therapeutic, so tackling those garden weeds may have more benefits than you think.
- Try yoga – it has a strong, relaxing, calming effect.
- Invest in a pedometer. This is a step-counting gadget that you can wear around your belt or waistband. You can use this to help you to gradually increase the number of steps you take daily.

Step 10: Enjoy your food

There are really no foods that should be totally avoided if you have diabetes or are trying to lose weight. Cutting out everything you enjoy can make you feel resentful and you will be more likely to give up on the whole plan. Do allow yourself small amounts of the foods you really enjoy, as a treat now and then. It may be a glass of fine wine, or a couple of squares of good chocolate or a meal out – enjoy your food.

Shopping and cooking for diabetes

When it comes to food shopping, the good news is that you only need to follow the same healthy-eating guidelines as everybody else. You do not need to buy special foods and don't need to shop at a specialist store. Everything you need for a healthy diabetic diet can be bought from your local shops or supermarket.

The healthy eating guidelines that the government recommend are listed below and show broadly what you should be aiming towards in your diet.

It's a good idea to keep the Dietary Guidelines for Diabetes (page 10) in your head when you go shopping because it will help you achieve a healthier selection of foods for the whole family. Concentrate on buying the healthier foods such as fruit, vegetables, seeded bread, wholegrain cereals, lean meat and reduced-fat dairy products. Choose fatty and sugary foods as occasional treats rather than as a necessary part of your diet.

Balance your trolley!

Another way to think about your diet when shopping is to divide your trolley up into five main areas: bread, potatoes and cereals; fruit and vegetables; milk and dairy; meat, fish, nuts and fatty and sugary foods. The illustration on page 24 shows the proportion of each foodstuff you should be aiming for.

Imagine your supermarket store is divided into these five sections and that your trolley contains foods roughly in line with the plate model. You could even try dividing your time in proportion too. For example, spend more time looking at the variety of fruit and vegetables and starchy cereals now available, and less time on fatty snack foods. This will help you make healthy choices and will also add variety to your diet. Some people find that shopping on the internet saves money and stops them buying foods from less healthy aisles, as they are not tempted by the smells of the bakery or the special offers in the cakes and puds section.

Fruit and vegetables

These provide valuable vitamins, minerals and fibre whilst being low in fat and calories, so try to include some at every meal. They also make great snacks. Fresh, frozen, canned and dried produce all count. Aim to eat at least five portions a day.

Bread, cereals and potatoes

Starchy foods such as bread, cereals and potatoes should make up the main part of most meals. These foods provide energy (in the form of carbohydrates), vitamins and minerals. Choose high-fibre, lower-GI varieties such as pasta if possible as these raise blood sugar levels more slowly.

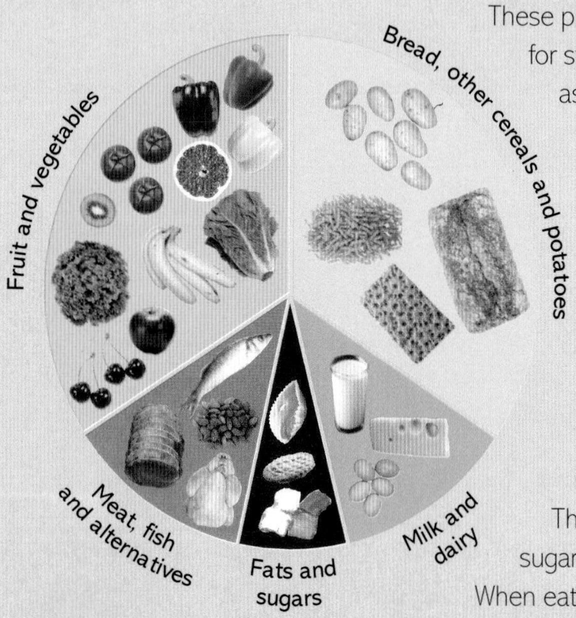

Milk and dairy foods

These provide protein and are a good source of calcium, which is necessary for strong bones and teeth. It's best to choose reduced-fat versions such as semi-skimmed milk and reduced-fat cheese. Aim to eat a moderate amount of these foods.

Meat, fish and alternatives

Meat, poultry, all fish, eggs, nuts and pulses are included here. They provide protein, vitamins and minerals, but you don't need large quantities. Aim for two to three portions every day and try to choose leaner cuts of meat. Include one portion of oily fish a week, which will provide beneficial omega 3 fatty acids.

Occasional foods

These include biscuits, cakes and pastries, which are high in fat and sugar, and not essential to a healthy diet, but add extra choice and interest. When eaten as low-fat, low-sugar treats, they can form part of a healthy diet, but don't go overboard! Choose low-fat low-sugar types and, if you do eat sweet foods, remember to have them at the end of a meal. The other ingredients of the meal will help to slow down the consequent rise in blood glucose, especially if you are eating lower GI meals.

The healthy fridge makeover

Keeping your fridge well stocked is essential so that you always have healthy food to hand and are not tempted to indulge in less healthy foods. The foods that have been highlighted in bold have a low GI and can therefore be useful in lowering the overall GI of a meal. Be prepared by having the following foods in your fridge:

- **Semi skimmed milk** – suitable for the whole family, except children under two years who need full fat milk. If you prefer, choose skimmed milk and be aware that this milk is not suitable for children under five.

Fruit and vegetables
Bread, other cereals and potatoes
Meat, fish and alternatives
Fats and sugars
Milk and dairy

Above: A balanced diet should be made up of these foods in these proportions.

Diagram reproduced with the kind permission of the Food Standards Agency.

- Cheese – opt for reduced or half-fat cheeses or cottage cheese which have less fat than standard cheeses. Buy cheese with a strong flavour to help you use less, which will save you calories and fat.
- Jam and marmalade – for a healthier alternative try the **reduced-sugar versions**, which taste just as good. Spread them on **grainy or seeded breads** to help lower the GI.
- Opt for reduced-fat dressings and mayonnaise. For sauces such as ketchup, reduced- sugar versions can be useful.
- Go for **plain yogurt and fromage frais**, adding fresh fruit such as **peaches, cherries and raspberries**. Or choose a **low-fat** or **diet yogurt** instead.
- Use a low-fat spread or one containing olive oil, which is high in monounsaturated fats and low in saturated fats.
- Use **diet mixers and low-calorie or diet soft drinks** instead of full-sugar versions.
- Choose **unsweetened fruit juices**. In between meals, these drinks can make your blood glucose rise quickly, so it's best to have them with a meal. This slows down the rise in blood glucose.
- Choose lean cuts of meat or ensure that excess fat is trimmed before cooking. Skim off the fat that has settled on top of stews or curries, and throw away the fat that has drained off a roast joint.
- Keep lots of **fresh fruit and vegetables** to hand as they're low in fat and calories. Fruit makes a great snack and vegetables can always be added to meals to lower the GI and help you reach your target of five portions a day.

The healthy storecupboard makeover

- **Pasta and basmati rice** are great storecupboard foods. They take very little time to cook and offer a low to medium GI.
- **Lentils and pulses** can be added to casseroles and stews to provide extra fibre and texture. They are available canned or dried.
- Ordinary baked beans do contain sugar, but they are also a good source of soluble fibre and consequently do not make your blood glucose rise as quickly as you might expect. Use a reduced-sugar version if you prefer.
- For breakfast cereals, opt for high fibre versions without added sugar. Check the label and compare brands. **Porridge oats** are fantastic, as are bran flakes and **muesli** – look for varieties with no added sugar.
- For bread it is best to go for wholemeal breads and those with **added grains or seeds,** which are digested more slowly. For a change, why not try **tortillas**?
- Choose plain biscuits, such as **rich tea and oatcakes**.
- **Canned fruit in natural juice** makes a healthier choice than fruit in syrup.
- To make quick desserts, keep sugar-free jellies and instant desserts. Also opt for **reduced-sugar custard** and **lower-fat rice pudding**.
- Cook with olive oil or rapeseed oil, as these are higher in monounsaturated fats.

Labels made easy

When shopping for healthy foods, the information on a packet can help you decide whether or not it is suitable for you. Products now carry a lot of information and knowing what you should be looking for and how to understand it can be daunting. Below is a typical nutrition information panel that you might see on the back of a product. It lists the main nutrients the food provides. Information is listed per 100g which allows comparisons to be made between products and also per serving which is more relevant as you rarely eat exactly 100g of a food.

A typical nutrition information panel

	Approx per serving (half a pot)	**Per 100g**
Energy	590Kj (122Kcal)	226Kj (54Kcal)
Protein	3.0g	1.3g
Carbohydrates	12.8g	5.7g
of which sugars	11.7g	5.2g
Fat	6.5g	2.9g
of which saturates	1.4g	0.6g
Fibre	2.0g	0.9g
Sodium	0.6g	0.3g
Salt equivalent	1.5g	0.8g

Whilst a nutrition information panel is useful, it is more relevant to relate the figures to how much of a nutrient you should be getting a day. This is where guideline daily amounts (GDAs, see below) can help. These provide a general idea about the amounts of nutrients you should be consuming in a day. GDAs only apply to adults and should only be used as a guide, as they do not take into account a person's body weight and physical activity levels.

By comparing the figures in the nutrition information panel above with the GDAs, shown below, you can get an idea how a serving of a product fits into your daily diet. The product is not contributing significantly to fat or calorie intakes, however the salt level (1.5g per serving) is fairly high, particularly for a woman's diet. (And in case you're trying to guess, it's a soup!) For the sugars the GDA is for 'added sugar'. From the nutrition

Guideline daily amounts

Nutrient	**Men**	**Women**
Calories	2500	2000
Fat	95g	70g
Saturated fat	30g	20g
Added sugar	30g	20g
Fibre	20g	16g
Salt	7g	5g

information panel it looks like the product is quite high in sugars but it is not clear whether the sugar is naturally occurring or has been added. This is where an ingredients list can help you find out more. Remember that sugar comes in many guises, such as honey, glucose syrup or dextrose. Another way of working out how a food might fit into your diet is to use the table below which aims to show how much of each nutrient counts as a little and a lot. This is useful for comparing products, and you can also use it when looking at the nutrition information panel.

	A lot (per 100g of food)	**A little** (per 100g of food)
Fat	20g	3g
Saturated fat	5g	1g
Sugar	10g	2g
Fibre	3g	0.5g
Sodium	0.5g	0.1g
Salt	1.5g	0.3g

'Better for you' foods

You may see products with healthy eating logos and nutrition claims on them, which are used to highlight and promote the product's nutritional benefits. When studying the claims, be cautious, as although the claims are legally defined, they can still be confusing and may not be as good as they first appear. For example, a product may say '25 per cent less fat' but if the standard product has 40g of fat, then the 'healthier' version will still have 30g of fat, which is still very high. Use healthy eating logos and claims as a way of spotting 'healthier' products, but do also check the nutrition information if you're not sure what the claims mean.

Cook your own healthy food

In this book you'll find a host of ideas on how to make your own recipes healthier. So when you try out a recipe, be aware of how the fat content has been reduced (for example, by using half-fat crème fraîche or Greek yogurt instead of double cream), or how the sugar has been lowered (by adding more fruit, for example). This will help you to build your own repertoire of recipes.

Enjoy different meal occasions and experiment with the varied ideas within these chapters. They range from special menu items for guests and formal meals, to more casual everyday dining. If you happen to choose a slightly more calorific course than you feel you should, simply team it up with fruit or low-fat yogurt rather than go overboard with one of the desserts. And it's good practice to get into the habit of accompanying all meals with steamed vegetables or salad (choose a fat-free dressing). This will help to fill you up and lower the overall GI of the meal. Remember that if you want to change your eating or lifestyle habits, it's best to do so gradually, and if in doubt, discuss this with your GP or dietician. For further information see page 138.

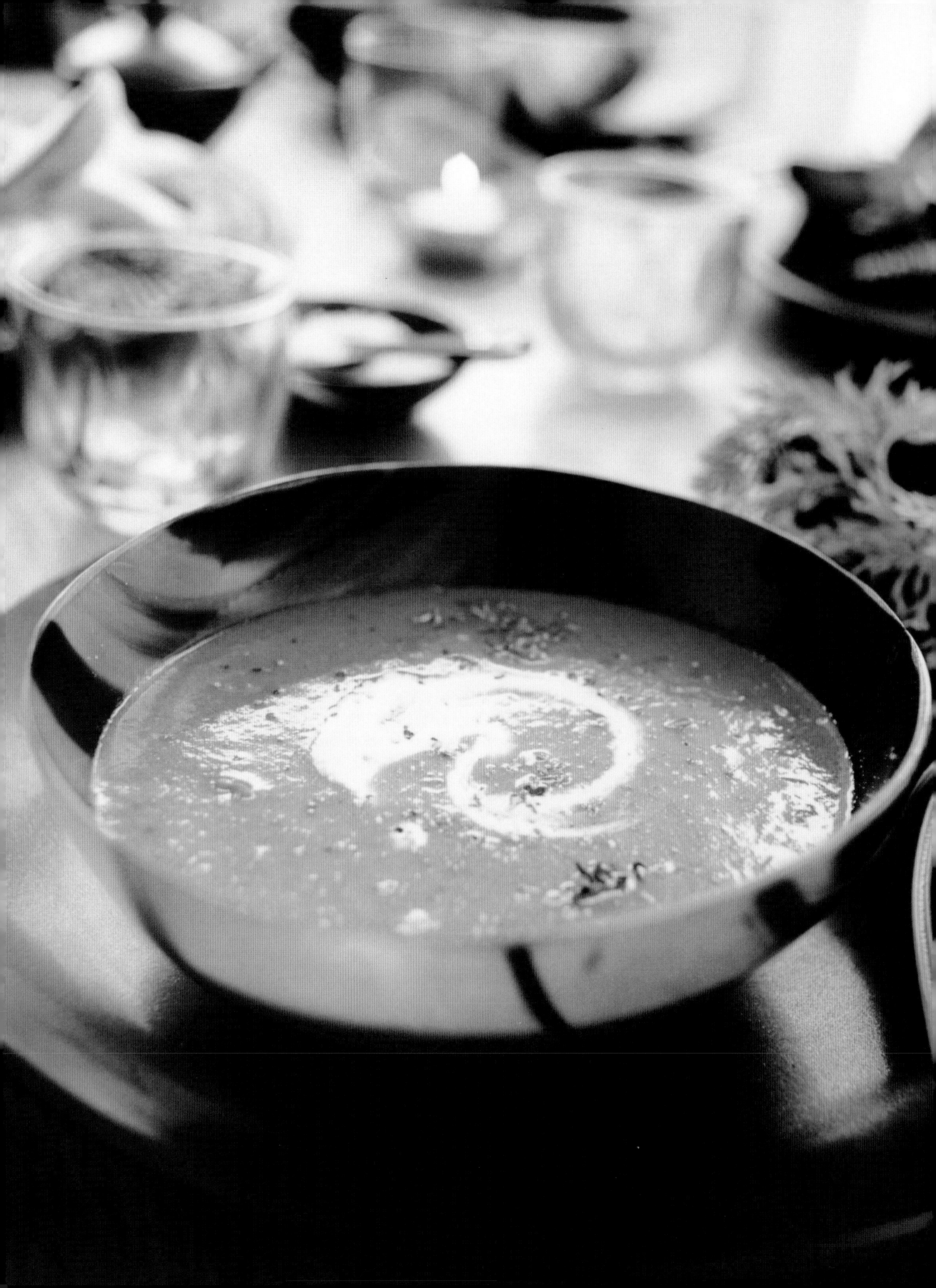

SOUPS

Herb and Lemon Soup

Chilled Tomato and Red Pepper Soup

Roasted Tomato and Pepper Soup

Smoked Haddock Chowder

Mexican Gazpacho

Courgette and Leek Soup

Cucumber, Yogurt and Mint Soup

Squash and Sweet Potato Soup

Mixed Mushroom Soup

Chunky Fish Soup

Herb and Lemon Soup

1.7 litres (3 pints) chicken stock
125g (4oz) orzo or other 'soup' pasta
3 medium eggs
Juice of 1 large lemon
2 tbsp finely chopped chives
2 tbsp finely chopped chervil
A few very fine slices of lemon to garnish

serves 6
preparation time: 10 minutes
cooking time: 15–20 minutes
per serving: 120 cals, 4g fat, 15g carbohydrate

A simple but sophisticated recipe for a smooth, light soup, with tiny pasta shapes and the delicate flavour of chervil and chives.

1 Bring the stock to the boil in a large pan. Add the pasta and cook for 5 minutes or according to the packet instructions.
2 Beat the eggs in a bowl until frothy, then add the lemon juice and 1 tbsp of cold water. Slowly stir in two ladles of the hot stock. Return the mixture to the pan, then warm through over a very low heat for 2–3 minutes.
3 Add the herbs and season. Serve in soup bowls, garnished with lemon slices.

NOTE: Don't boil the soup after adding the eggs – they will curdle.

Chilled Tomato and Red Pepper Soup

500g (1lb 2oz) ripe plum tomatoes
250g (9oz) sunblush tomatoes in olive oil, drained
100g (3½oz) marinated red peppers (preferably sun-dried)
2 garlic cloves, crushed
1 small red onion, finely chopped
6 tbsp sun-dried tomato paste
2–3 tbsp red wine vinegar
A pinch of dried crushed chillies
Dash each of Tabasco and Worcestershire sauce (optional)
600ml (1 pint) vegetable stock

serves 6
preparation time: 15 minutes, plus 4 hours (or overnight) chilling
per serving: 70 cals, 4g fat, 6g carbohydrate

Based on the Spanish classic, gazpacho, the traditional method of pounding the ingredients with a pestle and mortar is made much easier by using a blender. This is a recipe that actually tastes better if you make it ahead of time, as the flavours will develop and meld together while the soup is chilling in the fridge.

1 Put the plum tomatoes in a blender. Reserve six sunblush tomatoes, then add the remainder (drained) to the blender with the peppers, garlic and red onion. Whiz until smooth.
2 Add the tomato paste, vinegar, chillies, Tabasco and Worcestershire sauce (if using), and stock. Whiz briefly to combine. Season to taste with salt and freshly ground black pepper, and chill for at least 4 hours, or overnight.
4 To serve, spoon the soup into bowls, then garnish the top with a sunblush tomato and a basil sprig. Serve with fresh bread.

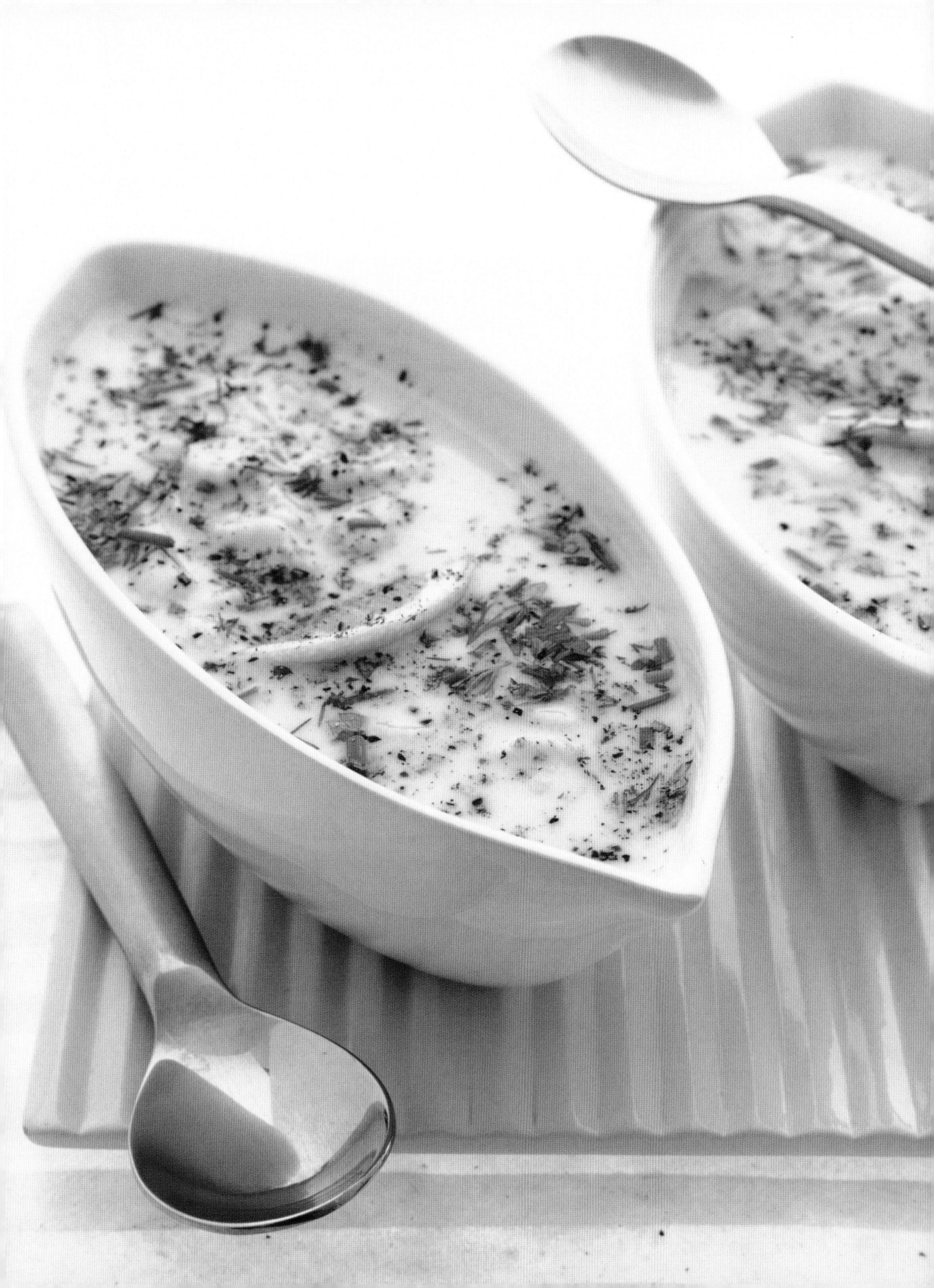

Roasted Tomato and Pepper Soup

1.4kg (3lb) full-flavoured tomatoes, preferably vine-ripened
2 red peppers, cored, deseeded and chopped
4 garlic cloves, peeled and crushed
3 small onions, peeled and thinly sliced
20g (¾oz) thyme sprigs
2 tbsp olive oil
4 tbsp Worcestershire sauce
4 tbsp vodka
Salt and pepper
6 tbsp half-fat crème fraîche

serves 6
preparation: 20 minutes
cooking time: about 1 hour
per serving: 170 cals; 8g fat; 16g carbohydrate

Tomato soup is one of the most popular of flavours. Once you've tried this version containing vodka, you won't want to eat tinned soup again!

1 Remove any green stalk heads from the tomatoes and discard. Put the tomatoes into a large roasting tin with the peppers, garlic and onions. Scatter 6 thyme sprigs on top, drizzle with the olive oil and roast at 200°C (180°C fan oven) mark 6 for 25 minutes. Turn the vegetables over and roast for a further 30–40 minutes until tender and slightly charred.
2 Put one third of the vegetables into a blender or food processor with 300ml (½ pint) boiled water. Add the Worcestershire sauce and vodka, plus plenty of salt and pepper. Whiz until smooth, then pass through a sieve into a pan.
3 Whiz the remaining vegetables with 450ml (¾ pint) boiled water, then sieve and add to the pan.
4 To serve, warm the soup thoroughly, stirring occasionally. Pour into warmed bowls, add 1 tbsp crème fraîche to each, then drag a cocktail stick through the cream to create a swirl. Scatter a few fresh thyme leaves over the top to finish.

Smoked Haddock Chowder

25g (1oz) butter
1 medium onion, finely sliced
900g (2lb) floury potatoes, peeled and cut into 1cm (½ in) cubes
½ a Savoy cabbage – about 450g (1lb) – sliced
900ml (1½ pints) semi-skimmed milk
2 smoked haddock fillets – about 300g (11oz) – skinned and cut into chunks
3 tbsp freshly chopped flat-leaved parsley

serves 4
preparation: 20 minutes
cooking time: 40–50 minutes
per serving: 330 cals, 7g fat, 44g carbohydrate

This warming recipe is a delicious combination of great flavours, including haddock and cabbage, and is perfect for a cold winter's day.

1 Melt the butter in a large pan, then add the onion and fry for 5–10 minutes until softened. Add the potatoes and cook over a low heat for a further 5 minutes.
2 Add the cabbage and stir in, then add the milk. Cover and bring to the boil, then simmer, partly covered, for 15 minutes until the potatoes are just tender.
3 Add the haddock to the pan and cook for a further 5–10 minutes. Stir in the parsley, season well with coarse black pepper and serve in warm bowls.

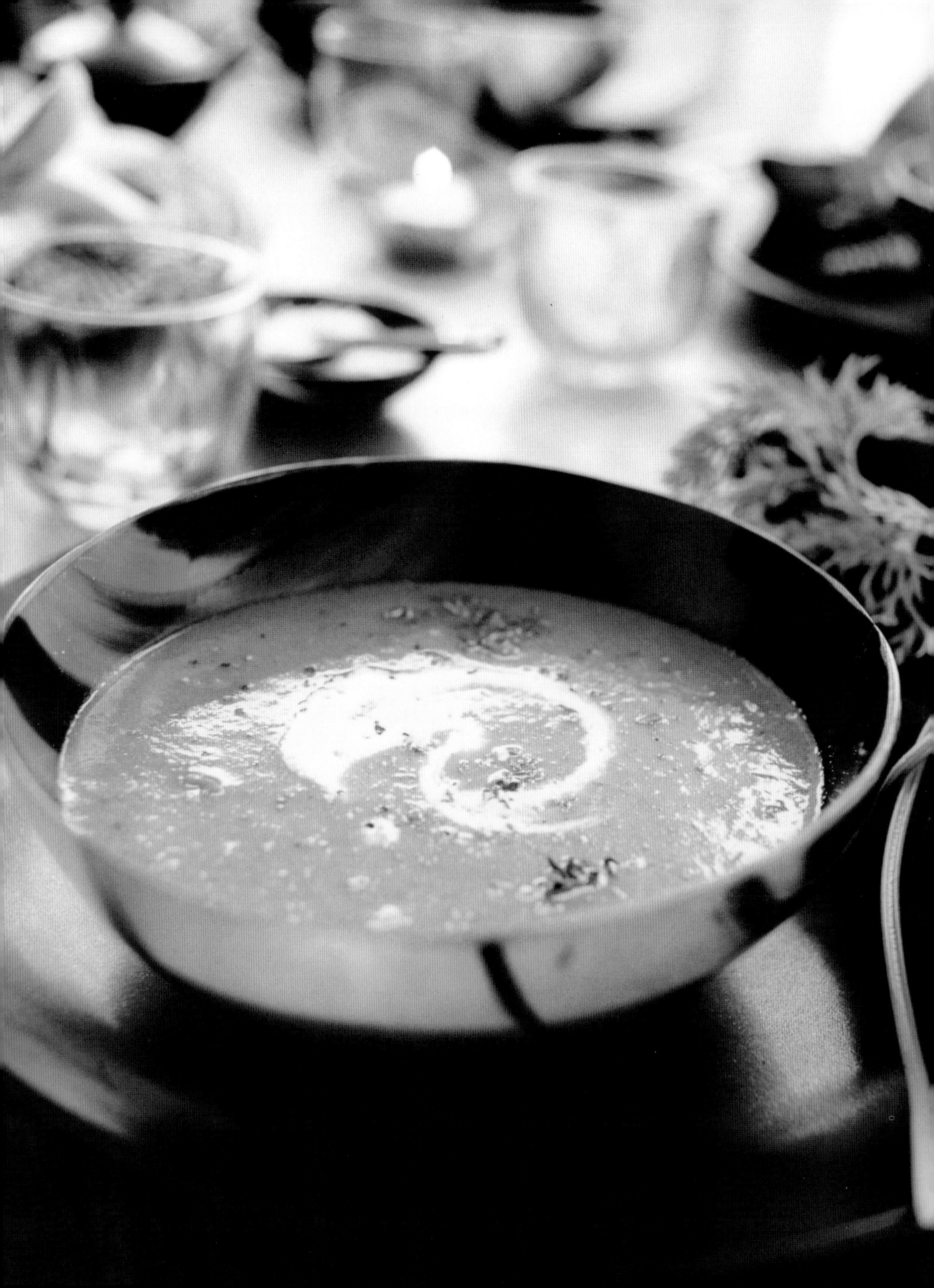

Mexican Gazpacho

for the gazpacho
900g (2lb) ripe tomatoes
4 garlic cloves
50g (2oz) fresh white breadcrumbs
3 tbsp extra-virgin olive oil
Juice of 1½ small limes
1 red chilli, deseeded and chopped
2 cucumbers, deseeded and chopped
2 bunches spring onions, chopped
1 red pepper, deseeded and chopped
600ml (1 pint) tomato juice
6 level tbsp fresh coriander leaves, chopped
to garnish
1 medium avocado
Juice of ½ small lime
142ml carton half fat crème fraîche (optional)
A few coriander sprigs

A thick, chilled tomato soup with the kick of fresh chilli. Make it a day ahead, if you can, and serve well chilled.

1 Score a cross in the skin at the base of each tomato, then put into a bowl. Pour over enough boiling water to cover them, leave for 30 seconds, then transfer to a bowl of cold water. Peel, discarding the skins, then cut into quarters. Discard seeds.
2 Put all the gazpacho ingredients into a big bowl and mix well, then whiz together in batches in a food processor until smooth and transfer to a bowl or jug. Season generously with salt and freshly ground black pepper and stir the soup well. Cover and chill for at least 2 hours.
3 Just before serving, peel and roughly dice the avocado, then toss in lime juice to coat. Serve the soup garnished with crème fraîche, avocado, a sprinkling of black pepper and coriander.

serves 8
preparation time: 25–30 minutes, plus 2 hours or overnight chilling
per serving: 180 cals, 12g fat, 13g carbohydrate

Courgette and Leek Soup

1 tbsp olive oil
1 onion, finely chopped
2 leeks, washed and sliced
900g (2lb) courgettes, grated
1.3 litres (2¼ pints) hot vegetable or chicken stock
4 short rosemary sprigs

makes 2.4 litres (4¼ pints) to serve 4 and freeze for 4
preparation time: 15 minutes
cooking time: 35–40 minutes
per serving: 50 cals, 2g fat, 5g carbohydrate

For maximum flavour, choose heavy, blemish-free vegetables. Use the whole length of the leeks – the white part gives a subtle creaminess while the green adds colour and punch.

1 Heat the oil in a large pan. Add the onion and leeks; cook for 5–10 minutes. Add the courgettes and cook, stirring, for a further 5 minutes.
2 Add the stock and three sprigs of rosemary, then bring to the boil. Season, reduce the heat and simmer for 20 minutes.
3 Cool the soup slightly. Remove the rosemary sprigs and whiz soup in a blender until smooth.
4 Cool half the soup and freeze (see below). Reheat remainder gently. Serve in warmed bowls sprinkled with the remaining rosemary leaves.

NOTE: The soup can be frozen in a sealed container and kept for up to three months. Defrost in the fridge overnight.

Cucumber, Yogurt and Mint Soup

1 cucumber, coarsely grated
500g (1lb 2oz) Greek-style yogurt
A generous handful of fresh mint leaves, chopped
1 large garlic clove, crushed
100ml (4fl oz) cold water or light vegetable or chicken stock
to serve
6 ice cubes
6 fresh mint sprigs

serves 6
preparation time: 15 minutes
per serving: 100 cals, 8g fat, 2g carbohydrate

This chilled soup is a favourite for summer – it's so very simple to make and incredibly refreshing. It works well with nothing more than a little water to thin it down (the grated cucumber will add more liquid) but tastes just that little bit better when you use some home-made chicken or vegetable stock instead.

1 Put all the ingredients in a large bowl and mix together. Chill until required.
2 Before serving, stir the soup, then taste and adjust the seasoning. Spoon the soup into bowls and drop an ice cube and a sprig of mint into each.

TESTER'S NOTE Sometimes cucumbers can be on the sweet side. After making the soup, taste it and add 1 tbsp white wine vinegar to balance the flavour if needed.

Squash and Sweet Potato Soup

1 tbsp olive oil
1 large onion, peeled and finely chopped
1–2 red chillies, deseeded and chopped
2 tsp coriander seeds, crushed
1 butternut squash, about 750g (1lb 10oz), peeled, deseeded and roughly chopped
2 medium sweet potatoes, peeled and roughly chopped
2 tomatoes, skinned and diced
1.7 litres (3 pints) hot vegetable stock
Salt and pepper

serves 8
preparation: 15 minutes
cooking time: 25 minutes
per serving: 100 cals; 2g fat; 19g carbohydrate

This is the perfect soup to prepare for guests on bonfire night or Halloween. It will ward off the cold all through autumn and winter. If you freeze on the day you make it, it can also be frozen for up to three months.

1 Heat the olive oil in a large pan, add the onion and fry for about 10 minutes until soft. Add the chillies and coriander seeds to the pan and cook for 1–2 minutes.
2 Add the squash, potatoes and tomatoes and cook for 5 minutes. Add the hot stock, then cover the pan and bring to the boil. Simmer gently for 15 minutes or until the vegetables are soft.
3 Whiz the soup in batches in a blender or food processor until smooth. Adjust the seasoning and reheat to serve.

Mixed Mushroom Soup

15g (½oz) dried porcini mushrooms
1 tbsp oil
1 small onion, chopped
450g (1lb) chestnut mushrooms, chopped
600ml (1 pint) hot vegetable stock
2 slices white bread, toasted
2 garlic cloves, peeled
Chopped flat-leafed parsley to garnish

makes around 1.1 litres (2 pints) to serve 4
preparation time: 15 minutes, plus 10 minutes soaking
cooking time: 35 minutes
per serving: 110 cals, 4g fat, 14g carbohydrate

Good, strong mushrooms are essential here. Chestnut can be replaced by large field mushrooms would work just as well.

1 Put the porcini into a bowl, pour over 75ml (3fl oz) boiling water and soak for 10 minutes. Strain the mushrooms, reserving the liquid, then roughly chop porcini, keeping 1tbsp to use as garnish.
2 Heat 1 tbsp oil in a pan, add the onion and porcini and cook over medium heat for 5 minutes. Add the chestnut mushrooms, turn up the heat and brown lightly for 5 minutes.
3 Add the porcini liquid and stock, then bring to the boil. Season well and simmer for 20 minutes.
4 To make croûtons, rub the garlic over the toasted bread to extract the essence of the garlic.
5 Cool the soup slightly, whiz in a liquidizer until smooth, then transfer to a clean pan. Gently reheat, then divide among four warmed bowls. Serve topped with the croûtons, reserved porcini and a sprinkling of parsley.

Chunky Fish Soup

1 grey mullet, Jamaican tilapia or red snapper fish (descaled, gutted, the head removed and reserved)
1 lemon
A few sprigs of thyme
2 garlic cloves, crushed
1 red medium or hot chilli, deseeded and chopped
1 level tsp paprika
1 bay leaf (optional)
250g (9oz) carrots, peeled and cut into large chunks
250g (9oz) potatoes, cut into large chunks
for the dumplings
75g (3oz) cornmeal
75g (3oz) self-raising flour, sifted
25g (1oz) butter, diced

serves 4
preparation time: 20 minutes
cooking time: 40 minutes
per serving: 300 cals, 6g fat, 43g carbohydrate

A restorative, cleansing, yet wholesome meal in a bowl that's great if you're feeling under par.

1 Cut the fish into four steaks. Put into a shallow dish and season generously. Squeeze over the juice from one half of the lemon and sprinkle with thyme, garlic, chilli and paprika. Cover and set aside.
2 Put the bay leaf and vegetables into a large pan with ½tsp of salt, plenty of freshly ground black pepper, the fish head, the juice of the other lemon half and 1.3 litres (2½ pints) cold water. Cover and bring to the boil, then simmer for 10 minutes.
3 Put the dumpling ingredients in a food processor with a generous pinch of salt. Pulse for a few seconds to create coarse crumbs. Add 1–2 tbsp of cold water and whiz again to form a firm mixture.
4 Add the fish to the vegetables, along with the herbs and any liquid. Simmer for 5 minutes. Roll the dumpling mixture into eight balls; add to the simmering soup. Cook, covered, for 10 minutes. Spoon into bowls to serve.

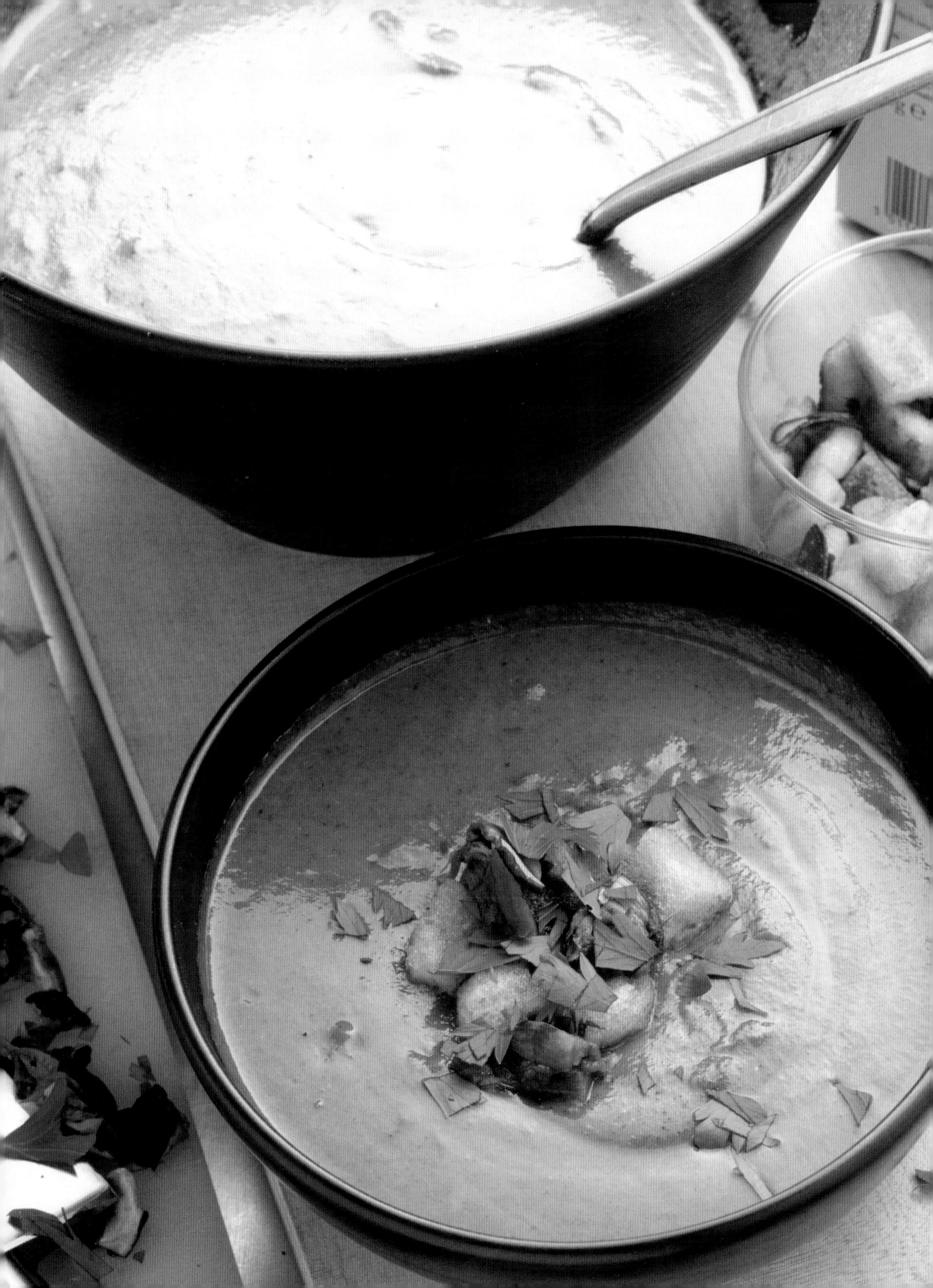

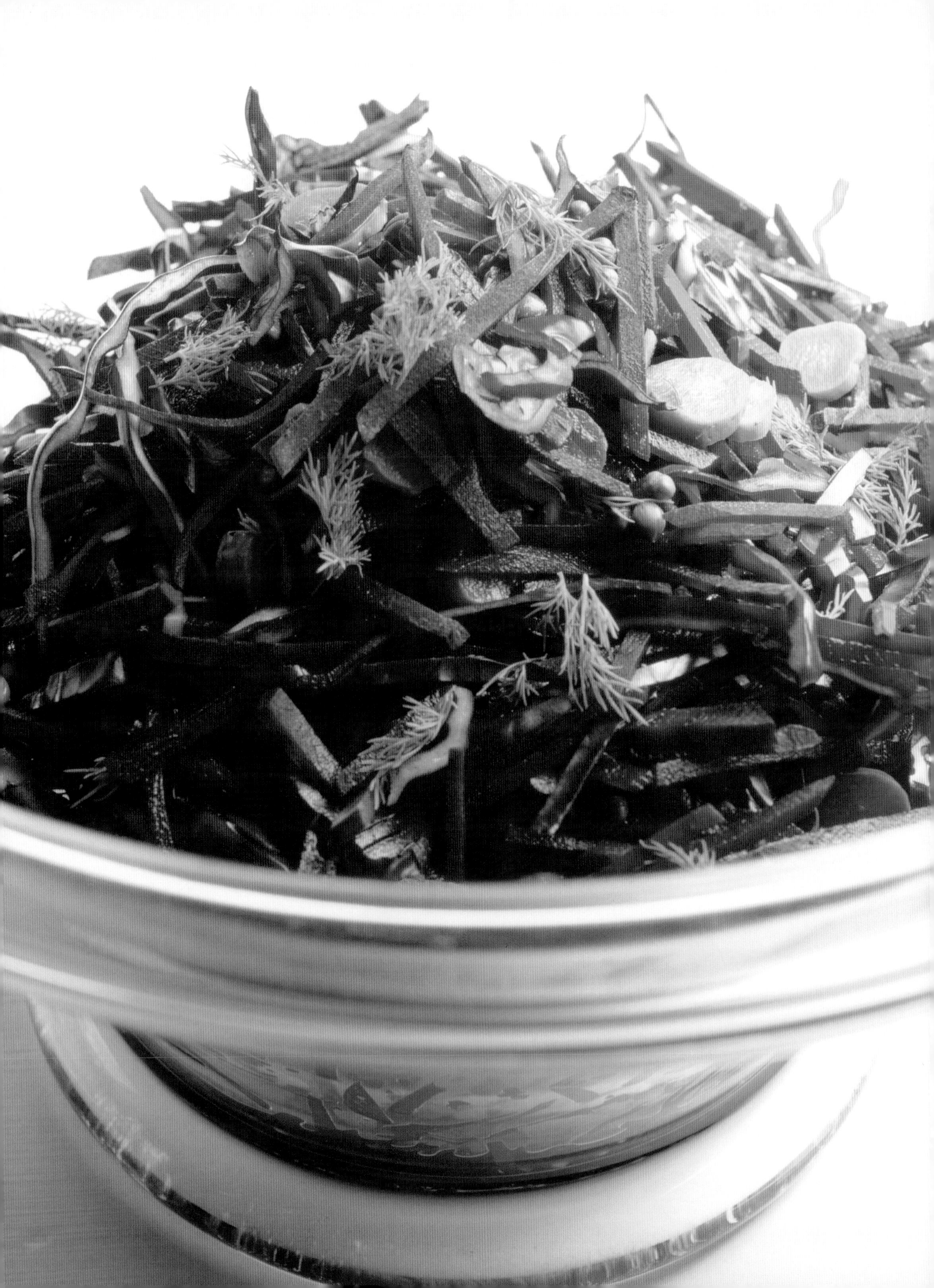

STARTERS

Wild Herb Kebabs

Bruschetta with Olive Tapenade and Antipasti

Peppers with Rocket and Balsamic Salsa

Red Cabbage and Beetroot Salad

Beetroot and Dill Salad

Pumpkin with Chickpeas and Tahini Sauce

Tomato, Mozzarella and Basil Salad with Balsamic Dressing

Saffron and Lime Prawns

Herbed Bulgur Wheat Salad

Rustic Bread with Tomato and Ham

Beef and Parma Ham Bites

Chickpea Salad with Lemon and Parsley

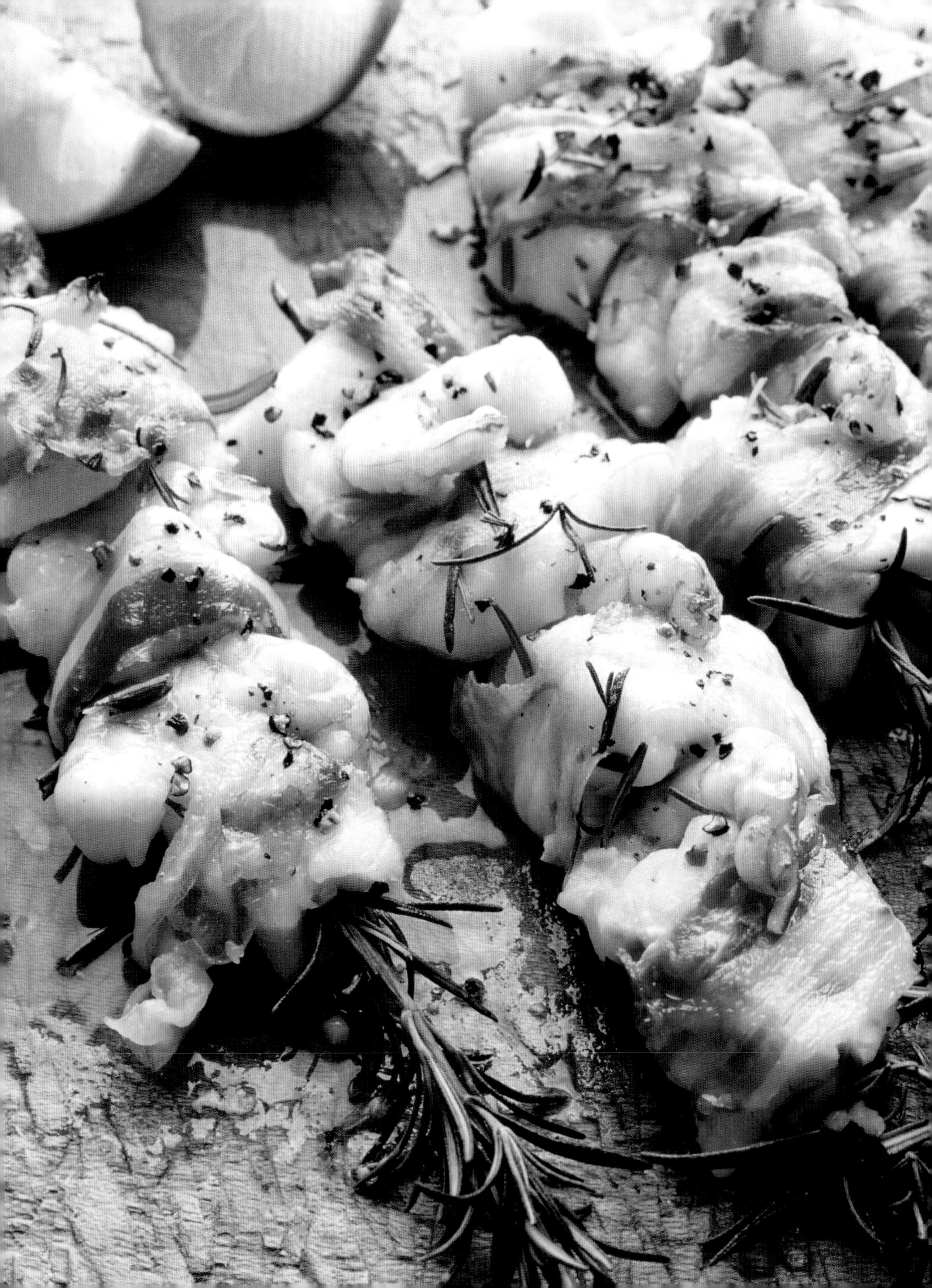

Wild Herb Kebabs

4 long, strong stalks of fresh rosemary
2 garlic cloves, crushed
2 tbsp olive oil
350g (12oz) firm white fish, such as cod, cut into bite-sized pieces
175g (6oz) large raw prawns, peeled
Zest and juice of 1 lemon
About 350g (12oz) tzatziki (if you can't find this ready-made, add chopped cucumber and fresh mint to low-fat natural yogurt, or use plain yogurt)
1 lemon or lime, cut into wedges, to serve

serves 4
preparation time: 25 minutes
cooking time: 10 minutes
per serving: 180 cals, 8g fat, 4g carbohydrate

Rosemary stalks are used in this recipe as skewers for the fish and shellfish, which leave a wonderful fragrant flavour.

1 Preheat the barbecue or grill. Strip almost all the leaves from the rosemary, apart from the top 5cm (2in). Roughly chop 2 tsp of the stripped leaves and mix with the garlic and oil. Stir in the fish, prawns, lemon zest and juice.
2 Cut the bare tip of each rosemary stalk to a sharp point, then use it to skewer the fish and prawns. Cover the exposed rosemary leaves with foil to prevent burning.
3 Cook the kebabs for 3 minutes on one side. Turn them over, remove the foil and cook for a further 3 minutes. Season and serve with tzatziki and lemon or lime wedges, with a green salad and couscous or new potatoes.

NOTE: If you can't find rosemary, use wooden skewers. Soak in cold water for 20 minutes before use to prevent them from burning.

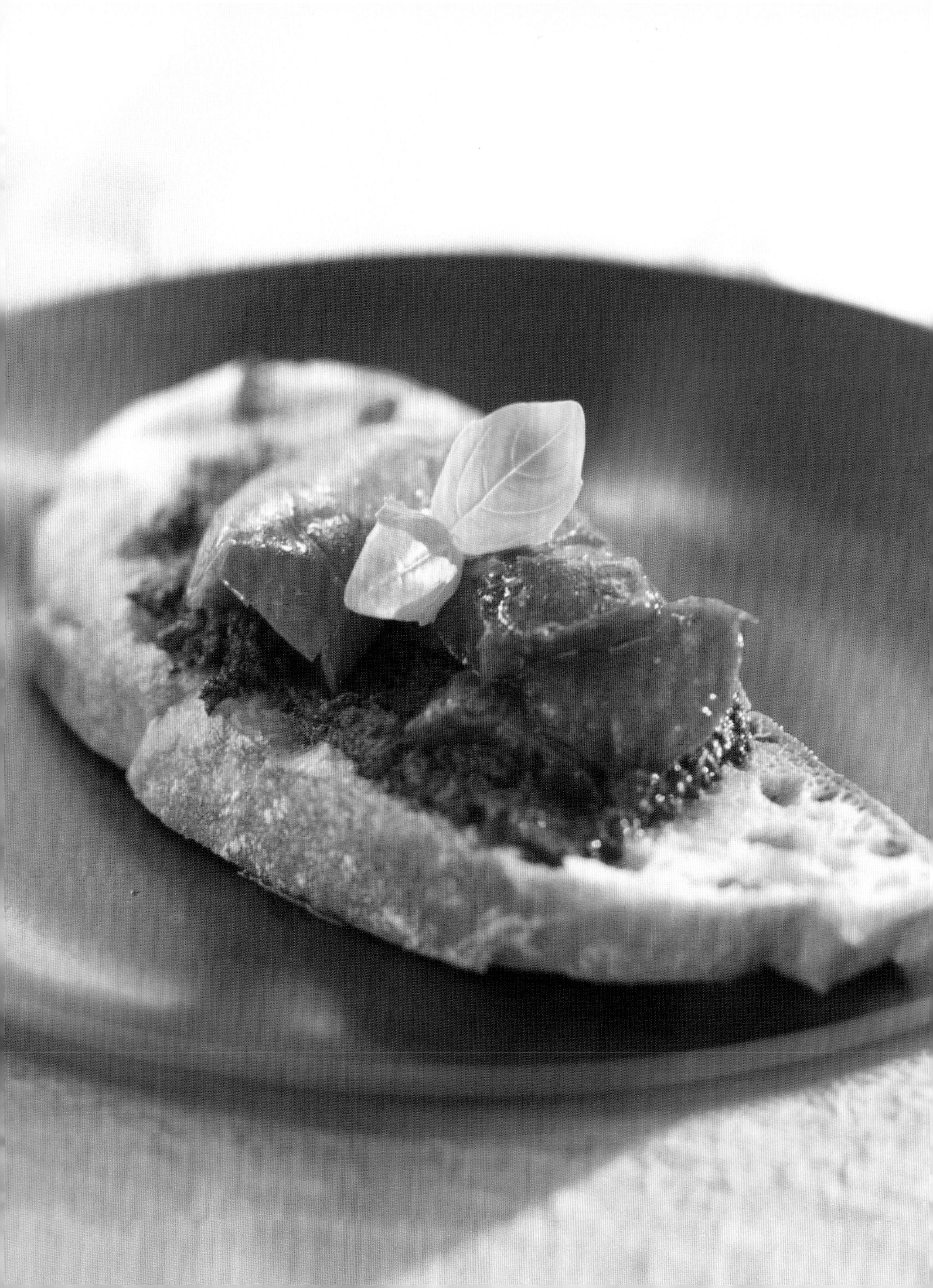

Bruschetta with Olive Tapenade and Antipasti

1 ciabatta loaf
A little olive oil to brush
Black olive paste (tapenade)
Selection of antipasti, such as marinated red peppers, artichokes and aubergines
A few basil sprigs to serve
Baby onions and aubergines

serves 6
preparation time: 5 minutes
cooking time: 5 minutes
per serving: 200 cals, 8g fat, 23g carbohydrate

These nibbles are ideal for dinner-party guests, and only take minutes to prepare.

1 Slice the ciabatta on the diagonal to make 12 slices and brush each side with olive oil.
2 Heat a griddle pan until hot and toast the ciabatta on each side.
3 Spread one side with olive paste. Let guests help themselves to the antipasti.

Peppers with Rocket and Balsamic Salsa

4 red peppers, halved and deseeded, each half cut lengthways into three
2 tbsp olive oil and spray oil
2 very large garlic cloves, sliced
1 small red onion, chopped
10 fresh thyme sprigs
3 tbsp balsamic vinegar
150g (5oz) sunblush tomatoes
50g (2oz) wild rocket

serves 5
preparation time: 15 minutes
cooking time: 40 minutes
per serving: 90 cals, 6g fat, 9g carbohydrate

Look out for sunblush tomatoes on supermarket deli counters – they're pricey but worth it. The tomatoes are slightly (but pleasantly) chewy, amazingly sweet and, best of all, ready to use, so you won't have to chop them up yourself.

1 Preheat the oven to 220°C (200°C fan oven) mark 7. Put the peppers into a roasting tin, then spray with spray oil and roast for 40 minutes until tender and slightly charred. After 20 minutes, push the peppers to one end of the tin and scatter the garlic, chopped onion and thyme at the other. Drizzle with 1 tbsp olive oil and roast for a further 20 minutes.
2 To make the balsamic salsa, pick the roasted thyme leaves from the stalks (discarding the stalks) and put into a small, screwtopped jar with the roasted onion and garlic. Add 1 tbsp olive oil and the balsamic vinegar. Season generously with freshly ground black pepper and a small pinch of salt, then shake well to combine.
3 Arrange the peppers in a large salad bowl, put the rocket on top, then scatter the sunblush tomatoes over. Drizzle with the balsamic salsa at the very last minute.

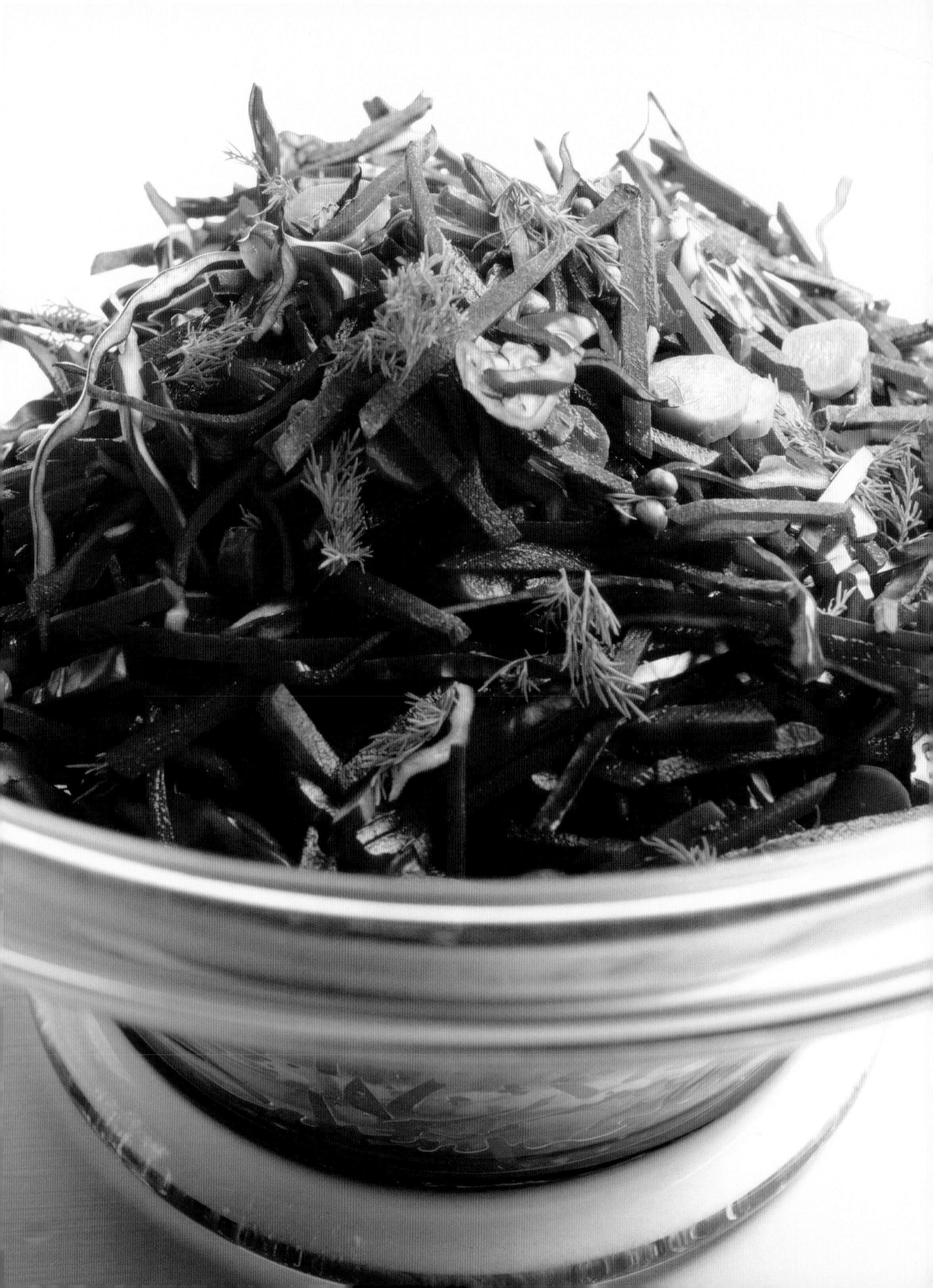

Red Cabbage and Beetroot Salad

½ red cabbage, cored
500g (1lb 2oz) cooked beetroot (see note)
8 cornichons (baby gherkins), sliced
2 tbsp baby capers in vinegar, rinsed
dressing
3 tbsp extra-virgin olive oil
2 tbsp sherry vinegar
3 tbsp chopped dill
Salt and pepper

serves 8
preparation: 15 minutes
per serving: 90 cals, 5g fat, 9g carbohydrate

Crunchy red cabbage, beetroot, cornichons and capers in a piquant dill dressing make an excellent starter or accompaniment to your main meal.

1 Finely slice the red cabbage and put it into a large bowl. Cut the beetroot into matchstick strips or grate coarsely, and add to the cabbage with the cornichons and capers. Toss well to mix.
2 For the dressing, put the olive oil, sherry vinegar and chopped dill into a small bowl. Season well with salt and pepper, then add a splash of cold water to help emulsify the dressing. Whisk together thoroughly.
3 Pour the dressing over the salad and toss everything together well.

NOTE: Buy vacuum-packed cooked beetroot or cook it yourself. Beetroot pickled in vinegar is not suitable. This salad is particularly good with baked ham.

Beetroot and Dill Salad

900g (2lb) beetroot
2 tbsp olive oil
Juice of 1 lemon
2 tbsp freshly chopped dill

serves 6
preparation: 15 minutes
per serving: 90 cals, 4g fat, 12g carbohydrate

Forget jars of pickled beetroot – the fresh version, cooked until tender, has an earthy flavour and a pleasant sweetness. Cutting into the bulbs makes them bleed furiously, so cook them in their skins before peeling.

1 Trim the stalks from the beetroot and discard, then rinse well. Put in a pan of cold salted water. Cover and bring to the boil, then simmer, half-covered, for 20–25 minutes or until tender. Drain well, then slip the skins off the beetroot.
2 Halve each beetroot and put in a bowl. Add the olive oil, lemon juice and dill, and season well with salt and ground black pepper. Toss together.

Pumpkin with Chickpeas and Tahini Sauce

900g (2lb) pumpkin or squash, such as butternut, crown prince or kabocha, peeled, deseeded and chopped into roughly 2cm (¾in) cubes
1 garlic clove, crushed
2 tbsp olive oil
2 × 410g tins chickpeas, drained
½ red onion, thinly sliced
1 large bunch coriander, roughly chopped

for the tahini sauce
1 large garlic clove, crushed
3 tbsp tahini paste
Juice of 1 lemon

serves 6
preparation time: 15 minutes
cooking time: 25–30 minutes
per serving: 210 cals, 12g fat, 18g carbohydrate

This is a warm, autumnal salad – which goes well with lamb. Tahini paste is made from sesame seeds and gives the dish a subtle, nutty flavour.

1 Preheat the oven to 220°C (200°C fan oven) mark 7. Toss the squash or pumpkin in the garlic and oil, and season. Put in a roasting tin and roast for 25 minutes or until soft.
2 Meanwhile, put the chickpeas in a pan with 150ml (¼ pint) water over a medium heat, just to warm through.
3 To make the tahini sauce, put the garlic in a bowl, add a pinch of salt, then whisk in the tahini paste. Add the lemon juice and 4–5 tbsp cold water – enough to make a consistency somewhere between single and double cream – and season.
4 To assemble, drain the chickpeas, put in a large bowl, then add the pumpkin, onion and coriander. Pour on the tahini sauce and toss carefully. Season with salt and freshly ground black pepper and serve while warm.

Tomato, Mozzarella and Basil Salad with Balsamic Dressing

2 tbsp balsamic vinegar
2 tbsp extra-virgin olive oil
25g (1oz) pine nuts
3 ripe beef tomatoes, sliced
100g (4oz) buffalo mozzarella, drained and torn into bite-sized pieces
15 small basil leaves

serves 4
preparation time: 15 minutes
per serving: 180 cals, 16g fat, 2g carbohydrate

This delicious salad only needs six ingredients and takes 15 minutes to prepare. Ripe tomatoes and soft mozzarella are drizzled with balsamic dressing, then scattered with toasted pine nuts and basil.

1 To make the dressing, put the balsamic vinegar and oil in a small bowl, whisk together and season generously with salt and freshly ground black pepper.
2 Put the pine nuts into a dry frying pan and toast, stirring, for 3 minutes. Set aside for a few minutes to cool.
3 Arrange the tomatoes and mozzarella on a large plate or shallow dish, season, and drizzle with the dressing. Scatter the pine nuts and basil on top and serve.

Saffron and Lime Prawns

8 bamboo skewers
Juice and finely grated rind of 1 lime
Good pinch of saffron strands
1 garlic clove, crushed
2 small red chillies, deseeded and very finely chopped
3 tbsp extra-virgin olive oil
32 raw tiger prawns, shelled

serves 8
preparation time: 10 minutes, plus at least 1 hour marinating time
cooking time: 4 minutes
per serving: 40 cals, 2g fat, 0g carbohydrate

Marinated in lime juice, saffron, garlic and chilli and quickly cooked, these tiger prawns make a mouthwatering starter.

1 Soak the bamboo skewers in water.
2 Pour the lime juice and rind into a small pan and heat gently. Add the saffron and leave to soak for 5 minutes. Stir in the garlic and chillies and add the olive oil. Pour into a screw-topped jar, secure the lid tightly and shake well.
3 Put the prawns in a shallow dish, add the marinade, cover and leave for at least 1 hour. Thread four prawns on each skewer. Put into a sealable container and keep cold.
4 To cook, lay the skewers on the grill (or barbeque) and cook for about 2 minutes on each side until they've just turned pink.

Herbed Bulgur Wheat Salad

175g (6oz) bulgur or cracked wheat
2 tomatoes, deseeded and diced
½ cucumber, deseeded and diced
2 shallots, peeled and chopped
4 tbsp chopped mint, plus leaves to garnish
4 tbsp chopped flat-leafed parsley
Salt and pepper
2 tbsp olive oil
juice of 1 lemon

serves 8
preparation: 10 minutes plus standing
per serving: 120 cals, 4g fat, 19g carbohydrate

Bulgur, or cracked wheat, has a lovely nutty flavour and should have a slight bite when cooked. Fresh herbs add depth of flavour.

1 Put the bulgur wheat into a bowl, pour on 300ml (½ pint) boiling water and cover. Leave to soak for 5–10 minutes until all the water is absorbed. Fork through, then set aside to cool.
2 Add the tomatoes, cucumber, shallots and chopped herbs. Mix well and season with a little salt and pepper to taste.
3 Add the olive oil and lemon juice and toss to mix. Leave to stand for a few hours if there is time, to allow the flavours to infuse. Garnish with mint leaves to serve.

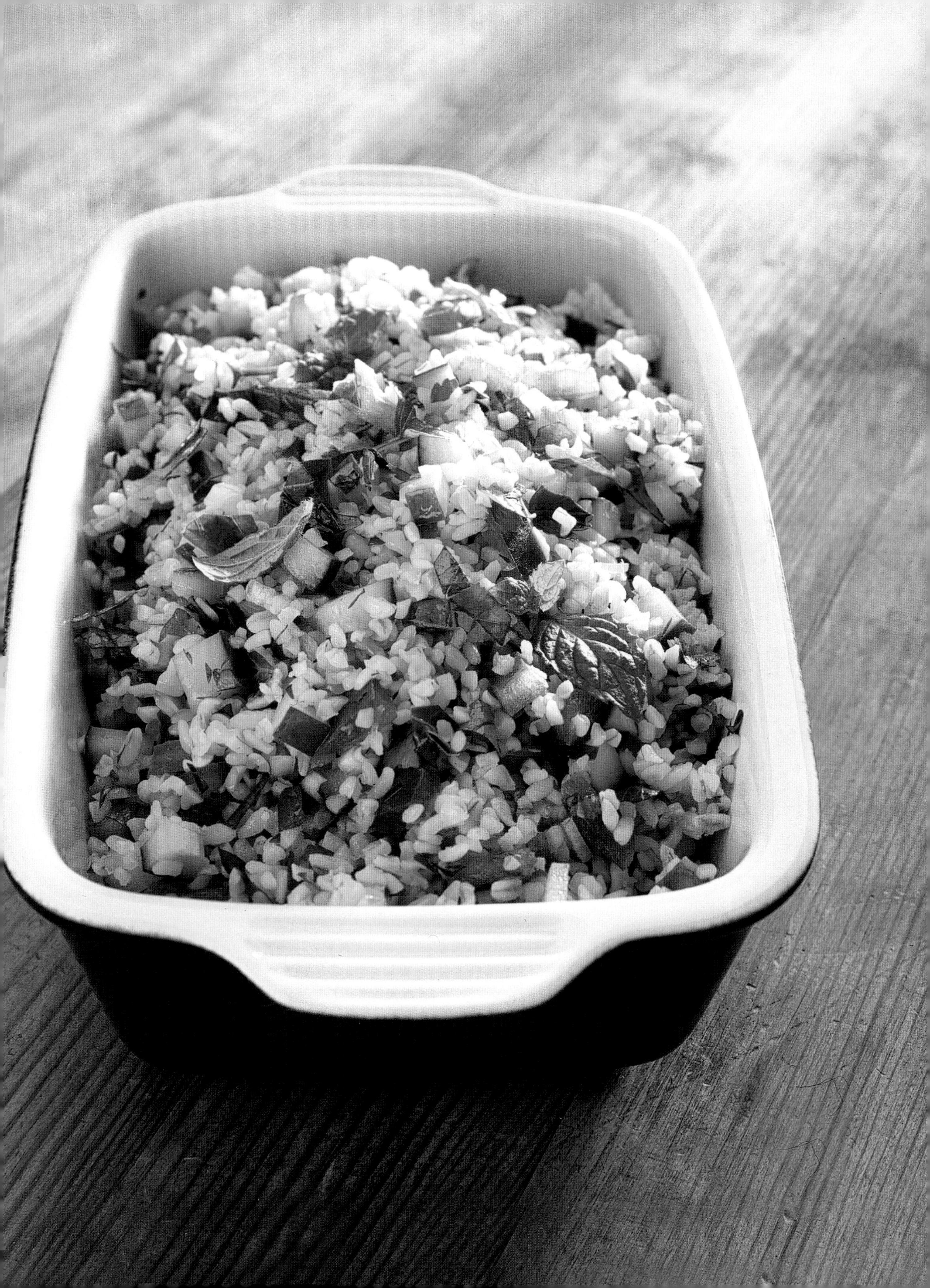

Rustic Bread with Tomato and Ham

4 slices country bread
A little Spanish extra-virgin olive oil
2 very ripe tomatoes, cut in half horizontally
4 slices Serrano ham

serves 4
preparation time: 5 minutes
cooking time: 5–10 minutes
per serving: 170 cals, 5g fat, 24g carbohydrate

In Spain, this is known as 'pan con tomate y jamón'. It sounds complex, but it's simply griddled bread rubbed with a juicy ripe tomato, topped with a slice of cured Spanish Serrano ham and drizzled with olive oil.

1 Heat a griddle pan. Brush both sides of the bread with oil and sprinkle a little salt over the top. Toast the bread on the griddle until golden.
2 Rub the cut side of half a tomato over one side of each slice of toasted bread to spread the flesh all over it.
3 Put a slice of Serrano ham on top of the tomato and season well, then drizzle with a little more oil and serve.

Beef and Parma Ham Bites

350g (12oz) fillet steak, about 2cm (¾in) thick
Salt and pepper
Olive oil, to brush
6 slices Parma ham
48 fresh basil leaves
24 sunblush tomatoes

makes 24
preparation: 15 minutes
cooking time: about 12 minutes
per bite: 30 cals, 1g fat, trace carbohydrate

Fillet steak, griddled and cut into cubes, then wrapped in Parma ham and basil and served on cocktail sticks with sunblush tomatoes and more basil – simple but delicious.

1 Season the steak all over with salt and pepper. Brush a griddle pan with a little olive oil, then heat over a medium-high heat. Add the steak and cook for 3 minutes on each side. Leave to rest for 5 minutes.
2 Cut each slice of Parma ham lengthways into 4 strips. Slice the steak into 4 lengths, then cut each into 6 pieces. Put a small basil leaf on top of each piece of steak, then wrap a strip of Parma ham around the steak.
3 Place the mini steaks on a lightly oiled baking sheet and roast at 200°C (180°C fan oven) mark 6 for 5–7 minutes until just cooked through.
4 Meanwhile, push a basil leaf and one of the sunblush tomatoes on to a cocktail stick and repeat until you have 24 assembled sticks. Take the baking sheet out of the oven and push one of the cocktail sticks halfway into each piece of beef, making sure the sharp end of the stick doesn't protrude. Serve at once, on warmed platters.

NOTE: Prepare to the end of stage 2 well in advance for convenience, and chill until ready to cook.

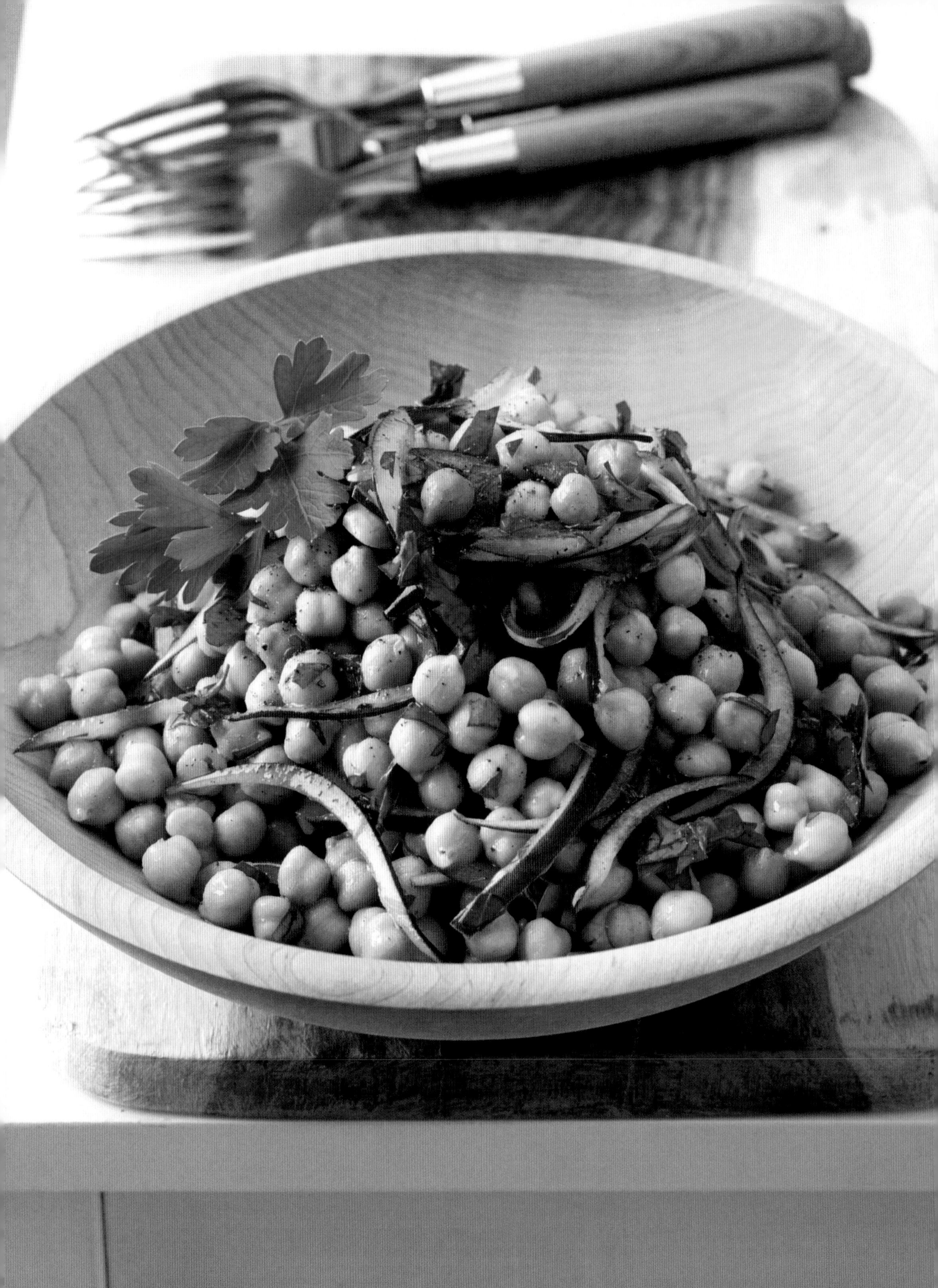

Chickpea Salad with Lemon and Parsley

2 × 410g cans chickpeas, drained and rinsed
1 small red onion, peeled and finely sliced
4 tbsp chopped flat-leafed parsley, plus extra sprigs to garnish
dressing
Juice of ½ lemon
2 tbsp extra-virgin olive oil
Salt and pepper

serves 4
preparation time: 15 minutes, plus standing time
per serving: 220 cals, 10g fat, 24g carbohydrate

Chickpeas and finely sliced sweet red onion, tossed in a zingy lemon dressing, make a delicious accompaniment to a summer barbeque.

1 First make the dressing. Put the lemon juice and olive oil into a bowl and whisk together. Season generously with salt and pepper.
2 Tip the chickpeas into a large salad bowl, add the red onion and chopped parsley, then drizzle over the dressing. Mix together well and check the seasoning. Set aside for 5 minutes to allow the onion to soften slightly in the dressing.
3 Serve the salad garnished with parsley sprigs.

NOTE: If you're making lots of salads, for a party, make this one the night before and store it, covered, in the fridge.

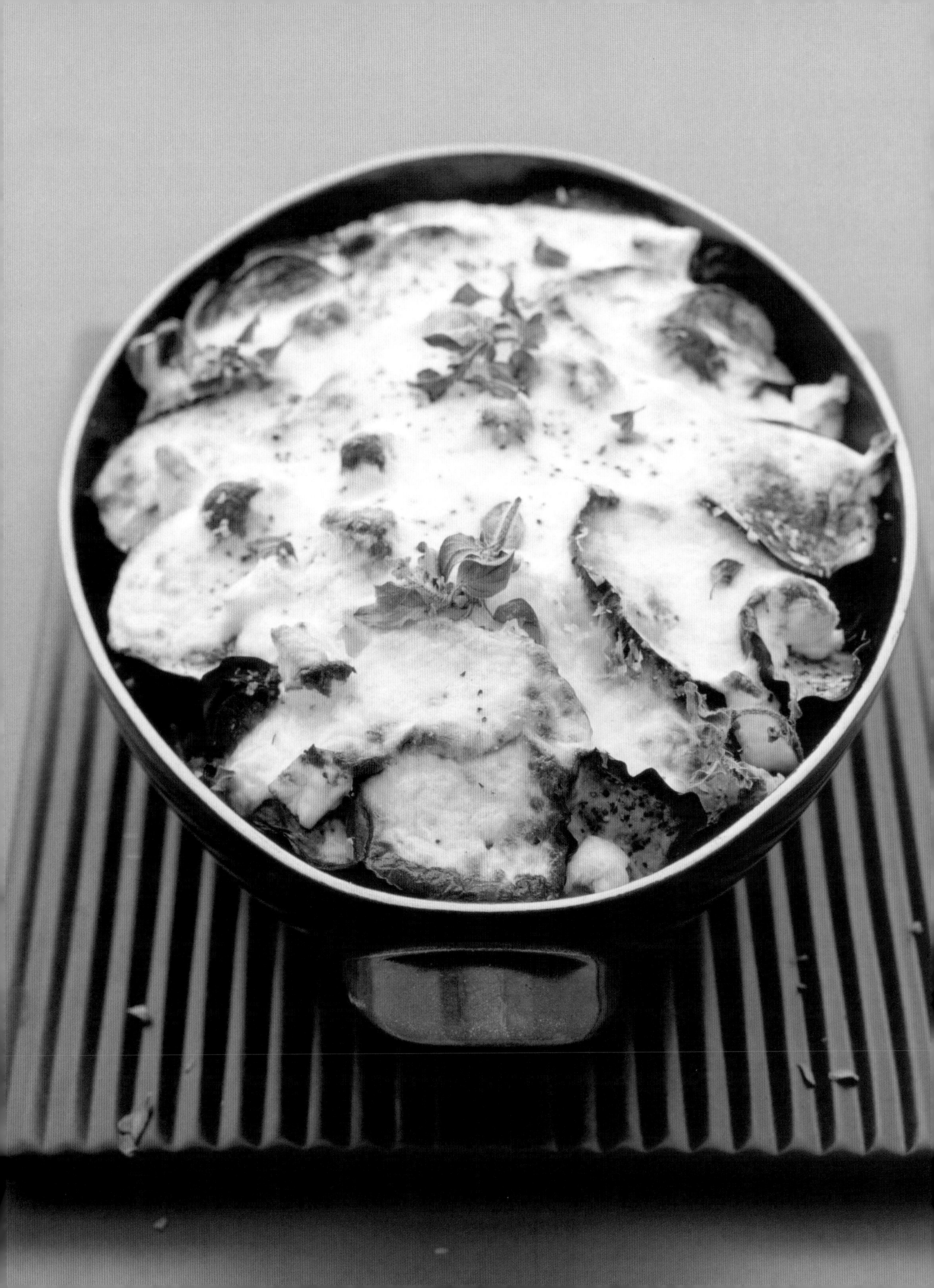

MEAT

Mustard Roast Beef

American-style Hamburger

Moussaka

Cottage Pie

Chilli Con Carne

Parma Ham, Courgette and Pine Nut Pizza

Garlic Soy Ribs and Sweet Potatoes

Cranberry and Orange Glazed Ham

Sausages with Roasted Potato and Onion Wedges

Pork and Vegetable Stir-Fry

Bacon and Cabbage with Parsley Sauce

Spicy Glazed Pork Chops

Pumpkin Mash and Sausages

Rack of Lamb

Curried Lamb with Lentils

Braised Lamb Shanks with Cannellini Beans

Moroccan Chicken, Squash and Chickpea Stew

Classic Roast Chicken

Crunchy Mangetout and tender Chicken

Chicken Curry with Rice

Turkey, Pepper and Haricot Bean Casserole

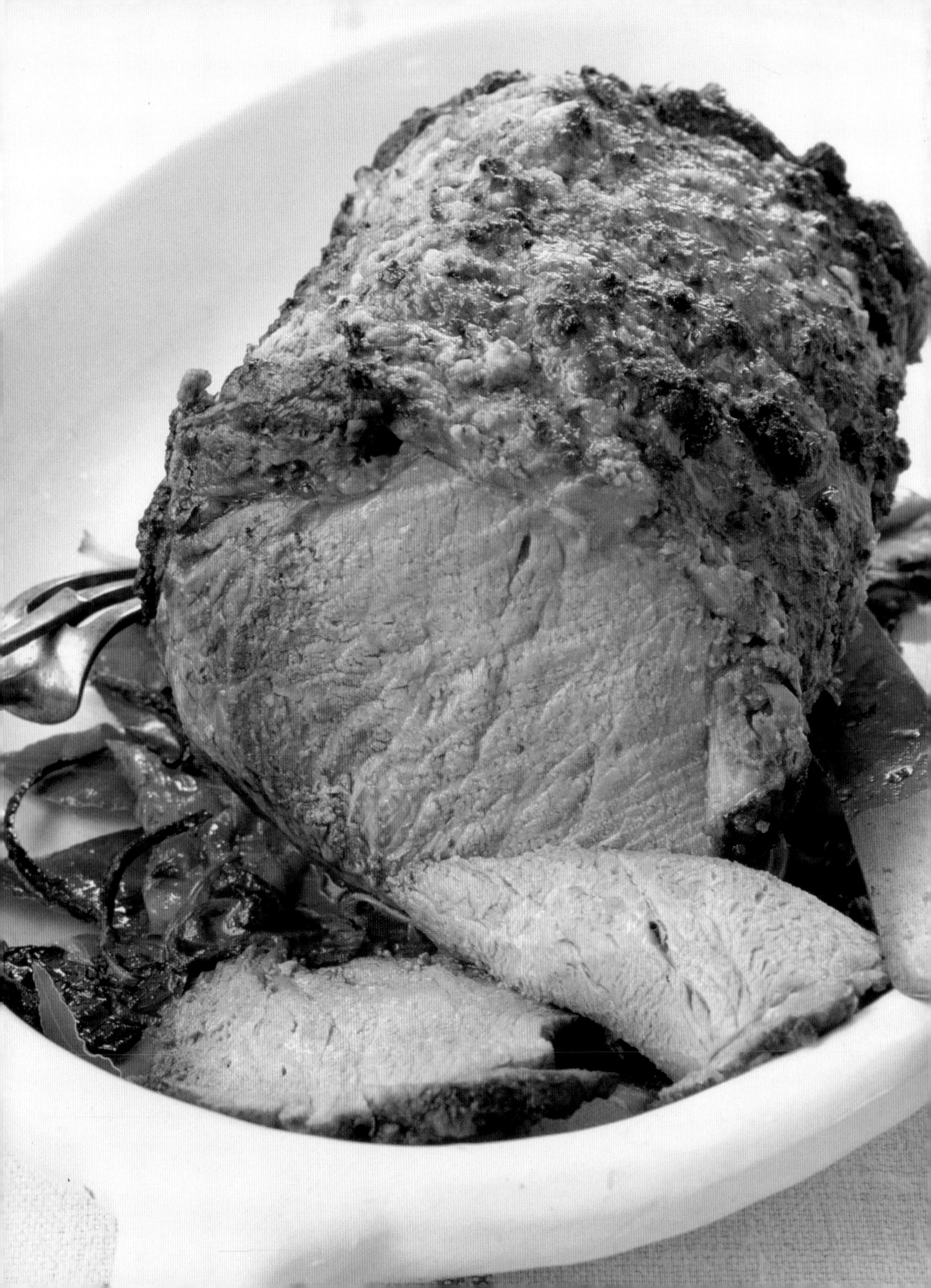

Mustard Roast Beef

1.1kg (2½lb) boned, rolled sirloin beef
1 tbsp olive oil
5 bay leaves
200ml (7fl oz) red wine
2 onions, sliced
2 tbsp English mustard
300ml (½ pint) vegetable stock, heated

serves 4
preparation time: 5 minutes, plus overnight marinating
cooking time: 50 minutes
per serving: 300 cals, 14g fat, 0g carbohydrate

A marinated joint makes an easy roast lunch. The marinade and the juices from the meat meld together for a delicious, no-fuss gravy. Serve with boiled potatoes and green beans.

1 To marinate the meat, put the beef in a bowl, add 1tbsp olive oil, five bay leaves, red wine, onions and marinate in the fridge for 4 hours or overnight.

2 Preheat the oven to 200°C (180° fan oven) mark 6. Put the joint in a roasting tin, scraping in all the marinade ingredients. Spread the mustard over the meat, then season well.

3 Add the hot vegetable stock. Roast for 15 minutes per 450g (1lb) plus 15 minutes (for a medium roast).

American-style hamburger

1kg (2¼lb) extra-lean beef mince
2 tbsp steak seasoning
Salt and pepper
A little sunflower oil, to brush

to serve:
6 large granary rolls
4 small cocktail gherkins, sliced lengthways
1 tsp American-style mustard
6 lettuce leaves such as frisée or batavia
4 large vine-ripened tomatoes, sliced
2 large shallots, peeled and sliced into rings

serves 6
preparation time: 20 minutes, plus chilling
cooking time: 15 minutes
per serving: 390 cals, 11g fat, 34g carbohydrate

Burgers are the ultimate fast food – but at their worst they can be unappetizing and full of fat. This home-made version, topped with crisp salad, makes an extra-lean gourmet sandwich.

1 Tip the beef mince into a large bowl and add the salt, steak seasoning, pepper and 2 tsp salt. Mix the ingredients together thoroughly, with clean hands.

2 Press the mixture into six lightly oiled 10cm (4in) rösti rings on a foil-lined baking sheet, or use your hands to shape the mixture into 6 patties. Cover with clingfilm and chill for at least 1 hour.

3 Heat a large griddle pan. Cut the granary rolls in half and toast, cut-side down, on the griddle until golden.

4 Lightly oil the griddle pan. Ease the burgers out of the moulds and brush lightly with oil. Cook the burgers over a medium heat for about 3 minutes, then turn carefully, using a palette knife. Put a few gherkin slices on each and cook for a further 3 minutes.

5 Spread the toasted side of the rolls with a little mustard. Put the rolls on warmed plates and cover with the lettuce, tomato and shallot rings. Put the burgers on top and sandwich together with the tops of the rolls. Serve straightaway.

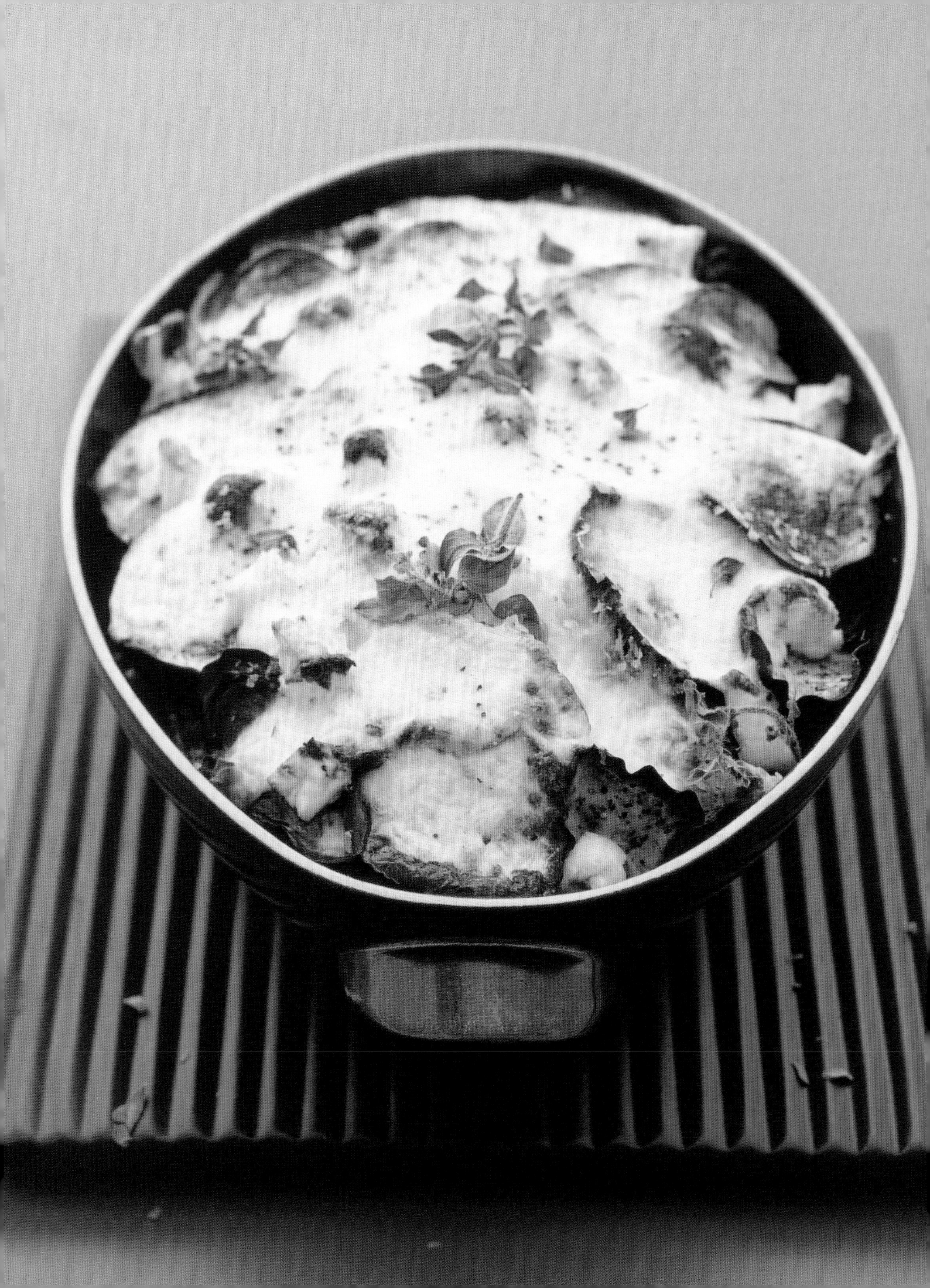

Moussaka

700g (1½lb) aubergines, trimmed and cut into 5mm (¼in) thick slices
3 tbsp olive oil
450g (1lb) onions, finely sliced
3 garlic cloves, crushed
700 (1½lb) lean lamb mince
2 level tbsp sun-dried tomato paste
400g can chopped tomatoes in rich tomato juice
1 cinnamon stick, crushed slightly
2 bay leaves
1 level tbsp freshly chopped oregano, plus extra sprigs to garnish

for the topping

200g (7oz) low-fat Greek yogurt
1 large egg
30g (1¼oz) freshly grated Parmesan cheese
A little freshly grated nutmeg
50g (2oz) feta cheese, roughly crumbled

serves 6
preparation time: 20 minutes
cooking time: 1 hour 10 minutes
per serving: 440 cals, 24g fat, 12g carbohydrate

This rich stew, made with a feta and yogurt topping, is a speciality of Greece and a great way of using aubergines while they're in season. To enjoy the dish at its best, eat it with a crisp salad.

1 Preheat the oven to 200°C (180°C fan oven) mark 6. Line baking sheet with foil and lightly brush the foil with 2 tsp oil. Arrange the slices of aubergine in a single layer on the foil, brush each side with a little oil, and season. Roast for 20–30 minutes, turning halfway through.
2 Meanwhile, heat the rest of the oil in a large pan. Add onions and cook over a low heat for 10 minutes or until soft. Add the garlic and cook for 2 minutes. Tip into a bowl while you cook the mince.
3 Put the mince in the pan and brown over a high heat. Return the onions and garlic to the pan. Add the tomato paste, chopped tomatoes, cinnamon, bay leaves and oregano. Bring to the boil and season. Simmer, covered, for 20 minutes.
4 To make the topping, put the yogurt, egg and half the Parmesan in a bowl. Season with salt, freshly ground black pepper and a little nutmeg, then mix everything together with a balloon whisk or wooden spoon until combined.
5 Put half the mince in a 2 litre (3½ pint) ovenproof dish. Add half the aubergine slices, overlapping where necessary. Season well and make further layers with the remaining mince and aubergine slices.
6 Top with feta, pour the yogurt mixture over and sprinkle with the remaining Parmesan. Cook in the oven for 35–40 minutes or until browned. Allow to cool for 10–15 minutes, garnish with oregano and serve.

TO FREEZE: After assembly, cool, wrap and freeze it will keep for up to three months. To serve, thaw overnight at a cool room temperature. Cook at 200°C (180°C fan oven) mark 6 for 45–50 minutes or until piping hot all the way through.

Cottage Pie

1 tbsp olive oil
2 onions, chopped
1 garlic clove, crushed
500g (1lb 2oz) extra-lean minced beef
2 level tbsp tomato purée
2 level tbsp plain flour
1 tbsp Worcestershire sauce
450ml (¾ pint) hot beef stock
2 bay leaves
for the mash
900g (2lb) potatoes, cut into large chunks
75ml (3fl oz) skimmed milk

serves 4
preparation time: 15 minutes
cooking time: 1 hour–1 hour 15 minutes
per serving: 420 cals, 10g fat, 53g carbohydrate

We've used less mince and more onions to make this traditional pie a healthier options. Better still, though, the basic recipe can be adapted easily for lasagne, chilli or a lightly spiced savoury bake.

1 Heat the oil in a pan and fry the onions and garlic gently for 10 minutes. Add the mince to the pan and cook on a higher heat, stirring constantly with a wooden spoon, until the mince is broken up and well browned.
2 Stir in the tomato purée and flour and cook for 1 minute. Add the Worcestershire sauce, stock and bay leaves. Cover, bring to the boil and season generously. Reduce the heat and simmer for 30–40 minutes until the meat is tender. Remove the bay leaves and discard, then spoon the mixture into a 1.8 litre (3¼ pint) ovenproof dish.
3 Meanwhile, cook the potatoes in a large pan of boiling, salted water. Drain well, tip the potatoes back into the pan and heat for 1 minute to dry off. Add the skimmed milk, season with salt and freshly ground black pepper and mash well. Preheat the oven to 200°C (180°C fan oven) mark 6.
4 Spoon the mash on top of the mince, spread over evenly and rough up the surface with a fork. Put the dish on a baking sheet to catch any spillages and cook for 20–25 minutes until golden and bubbling.

Chilli Con Carne

2 tbsp olive oil
2 onions, finely chopped
2 large garlic cloves, crushed
2 red chillies, deseeded and finely chopped
900g (2lb) lean minced beef
1½ level tsp hot chilli powder
1 level tsp ground cumin
1 level tbsp tomato purée
2 level tsp soft dark brown sugar
1 tbsp Worcestershire sauce
300ml (½ pint) beef stock
2 × 400g can chopped tomatoes
400g can red kidney beans, drained and rinsed
1tbsp freshly chopped flat-leafed parsley

Making double quantities of chilli means you can serve half with rice today and freeze the rest for a chilli bake next week.

1 Heat the oil in a large flameproof casserole or heavy-based pan, then add the onions, garlic and chillies and cook for 4–5 minutes until the onion softens. Increase the heat, add the beef and stir-fry for 5–6 minutes until browned all over.
2 Add the chilli powder, cumin and tomato purée and cook, stirring, for 1 minute. Add the sugar, Worcestershire sauce, stock and tomatoes. Bring to the boil, then lower the heat, cover and simmer for 30 minutes.
3 Add the kidney beans to the casserole and simmer for a further 10 minutes. Put half the chilli con carne aside and leave to cool. Garnish the remaining chilli with parsley, then serve with rice. Freeze the cooled chilli.

serves 4
preparation time: 20 minutes
cooking time: 55 minutes–1 hour
per serving: 240 cals, 9g fat, 14g carbohydrate

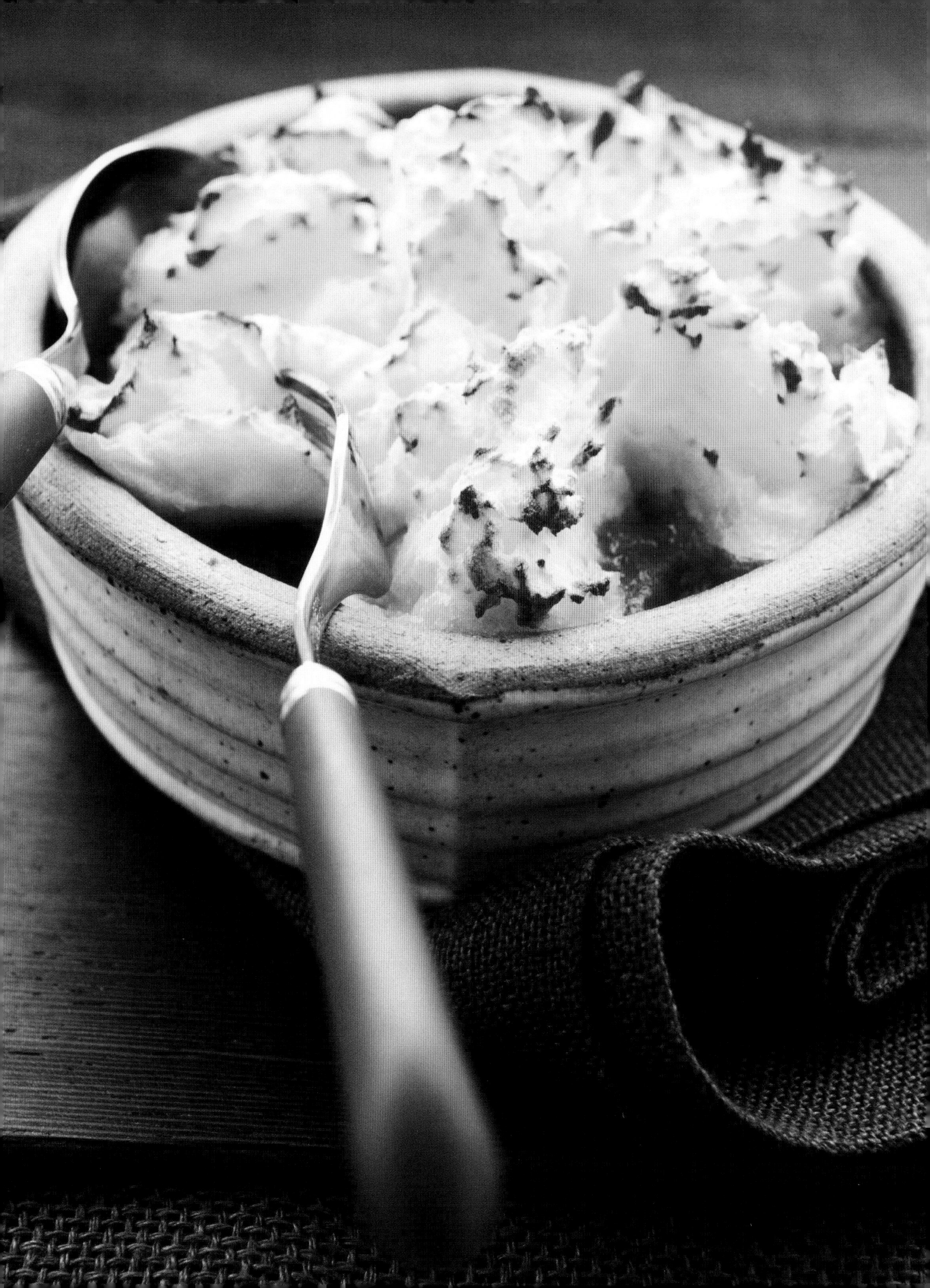

Parma Ham, Courgette and Pine Nut Pizza

1 part-baked ciabatta loaf
250g (9oz) jar thick tomato and herb sauce
1 medium courgette
50g (2oz) Parma ham, torn into pieces
25g (1oz) pine nuts
50g (2oz) Parmesan cheese shavings

serves 4
preparation time: 10 minutes
cooking time: 10–12 minutes
per serving: 330 cals, 16g fat, 32g carbohydrate

Part-baked ciabatta bread makes an instant light, airy pizza base for these inspired topping ingredients.

1 Preheat the oven to 200°C (180°C fan oven) mark 6. Using a serrated knife, split the ciabatta in half lengthways, then put it on a baking sheet, cut-side up.
2 Divide the tomato sauce between the two halves and spread evenly on the bread. Trim the ends off the courgette, then run a peeler down the length of the courgette to make wide ribbons.
3 Arrange slices of courgette and ham alternately on top of the tomato sauce on both pizza bases. Scatter each with the pine nuts. Bake for 10–12 minutes until the topping is hot but not browned. Remove from the oven, scatter with the Parmesan, and season with salt and pepper. Serve with rocket leaves.

NOTE: Put a non-stick Teflon liner (available from most supermarkets) on top of your baking sheet to catch any spills such as melting cheese and save you time on the washing-up.

Garlic Soy Ribs with Sweet Potatoes

450g (1lb) rack of pork ribs, cut in half
½ lemon
1 level tbsp chicken seasoning
4 tbsp soy sauce
3 tbsp malt vinegar
3 level tbsp light muscovado sugar
2 garlic cloves, crushed
½tsp freshly grated ginger
1 tsp Chipotle Tabasco (if you have only the regular variety, just add a couple of drops)
125ml (4fl oz) beef stock, cooled
4 sweet potatoes, scrubbed
4 tbsp Greek yogurt
2 spring onions, trimmed and roughly chopped

serves 4
preparation time: 15 minutes
cooking time: 55 minutes
per serving: 440 cals, 17g fat, 49g carbohydrate

American restaurants may well serve each customer a whole rack of ribs – because ribs are the kind of thing you can eat and eat until you feel you're going to pop. But if you serve each person a generous baked sweet potato as well, one rack of ribs will be ample for four.

1 Put the rack of pork ribs into a shallow dish. Rub the lemon half over the meat, squeezing out the juice as you go, then sprinkle over the chicken seasoning, soy sauce, vinegar, sugar, garlic, ginger and Tabasco. Turn the ribs to coat evenly in the marinade. If you have time, cover and chill to marinate for at least 2 hours.
2 Preheat the oven to 200°C (180°C fan oven) mark 6. Put the ribs and marinade into a roasting tin and pour over the beef stock. Roast for 50–55 minutes, turning the ribs during cooking to coat in the sauce.
3 Meanwhile, wrap the sweet potatoes in foil and bake for 50–55 minutes until they are just tender. To serve, slash the top of each potato and squeeze the sides to push up the sweet flesh. Top each with a dollop of Greek yogurt and sprinkle with the spring onions. Cut between the ribs to separate them and serve alongside the sweet potato.

NOTE: To enhance the flavour of the sweet potatoes, drizzle with a little olive oil, then sprinkle the skins with sea salt before wrapping in foil and baking.

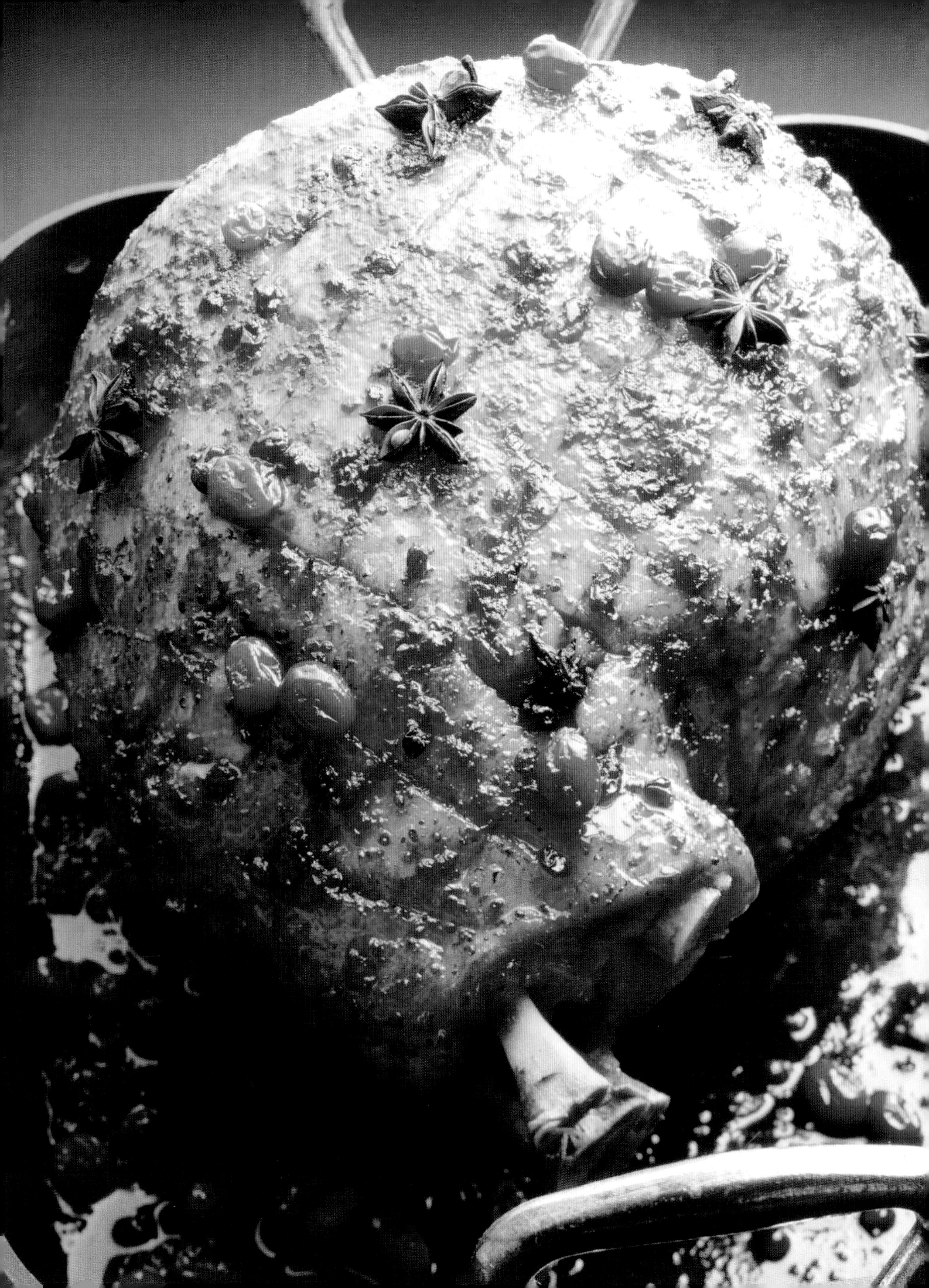

Cranberry and Orange Glazed Ham

4.5kg (10lb) smoked gammon joint, on the bone
2 celery sticks, roughly chopped
1 onion, peeled and quartered
1 carrot, peeled and roughly chopped
1 level tsp black peppercorns
Grated zest and juice of 1 orange
1 level tbsp light muscovado sugar
4 level tbsp cranberry sauce
1 level tbsp grainy mustard
50ml (2fl oz) cider
10 whole star anise
125g (4oz) cranberries

serves 16
preparation time: 15 minutes
cooking time: around 4 hours 20 minutes
per serving: 210 cals, 7g fat, 2g carbohydrate

Cranberry sauce, cider and orange juice combine in a glaze to give this ham a delicious flavour. Taste the stock once the ham is cooked at the end of step 1 – if it's not too salty, it makes a great base for soup. Just freeze for future use.

1 Put the gammon in a large pan, add the celery, onion, carrot and peppercorns, cover with cold water and bring to the boil. Simmer, covered, for 20 minutes per 450g (1lb) plus 20 minutes if the joint is 4.5kg (10lb) or less. If the joint is more than 4.5kg (10lb), simmer for 15–20 minutes per 450g (1lb) plus 15 minutes. Towards the end of the cooking time, preheat the oven to 200°C (180°C fan oven) mark 6.
2 Meanwhile, make the glaze. Put the orange zest and juice, cranberry sauce, mustard, cider and sugar in a bowl and stir everything together. Put aside to allow the sugar to dissolve. Season well with salt and freshly ground black pepper.
3 Lift the gammon out of the pan and put in a roasting tin. Leave to cool slightly. Using a sharp knife, remove the rind, leaving a layer of fat on the ham, and discard. Score the fat in a crisscross pattern and push the star anise into the fat. Spoon the glaze all over the joint. Roast for 15–20 minutes. Add the cranberries to the pan and baste the meat with the juices, then roast for a further 15–20 minutes, until deep golden. Serve hot or cold, carved into thin slices.

Sausages with Roasted Potato and Onion Wedges

900g (2lb) Desirée potatoes, scrubbed and cut into wedges
2 tbsp olive oil
3–4 sprigs rosemary (optional)
2 red onions, each cut into 8 wedges
8 lower fat sausages
100ml (4fl oz) chicken or vegetable stock

serves 4
preparation time: 10 minutes
cooking time: 1 hour 20 minutes
per serving: 470 cals, 20g fat, 55g carbohydrate

This doesn't take long to prepare – just chop everything and then let the oven do the work for you. Delicious, when served with a tomato chutney.

1 Preheat the oven to 220°C (200°C fan oven) mark 7. Put the potatoes in the roasting tin – they should sit in one layer. Drizzle over the oil and season with salt and freshly ground black pepper. Toss well to coat the potatoes in oil, then put the rosemary on top (if using) and roast in the oven for 20 minutes.
2 Remove the roasting tin from the oven and add the onion wedges. Toss again to coat the onions and turn the potatoes. Put the sausages in between the potatoes and onions. Return the tin to the oven for 30 minutes. Turn the ingredients with a fish slice, add the stock and cook for a further 20–30 minutes until cooked through.
3 Divide between four plates and serve immediately.

Pork and Vegetable Stir-fry

450g (1lb) pork fillet (tenderloin)
2 tbsp dry sherry
2 tbsp light soy sauce
2 garlic cloves, peeled and crushed
5cm (2 in) piece fresh root ginger, grated
1 tsp cornflour
1 tbsp groundnut oil
1 large carrot, peeled and cut into fine matchsticks
225g (8oz) broccoli, broken into small florets
8 spring onions, trimmed and finely shredded
150g (5oz) beansprouts
Salt and pepper

serves 4
preparation time: 15 minutes, plus marinating
cooking time: 15 minutes
per serving: 250 cals, 12g fat, 6g carbohydrate

Stir-frying is a great way to eat healthily, as cooking briefly over a high heat retains as many nutrients as possible. Use groundnut oil as it has virtually no flavour.

1 Trim any fat off the pork and cut the meat into thin slices. Put 1tbsp sherry, 1 tbsp soy sauce, the garlic, ginger and cornflour into a large bowl and mix well to make a marinade. Add the pork and toss well, then set aside for 15 minutes.
2 Heat a non-stick wok until very hot, then add the groundnut oil. Stir-fry the pork slices in two batches until browned; remove and set aside.
3 Reheat the wok, then add the carrot and broccoli, and stir-fry for 5 minutes. Add the remaining sherry and soy sauce together with 4tbsp cold water, and bring to just boiling. Add the cooked pork and stir-fry for 2–3 minutes to heat through.
4 Add the spring onions and beansprouts and stir-fry for 1 minute. Season with salt and pepper to taste, and serve with plain boiled rice or egg noodles.

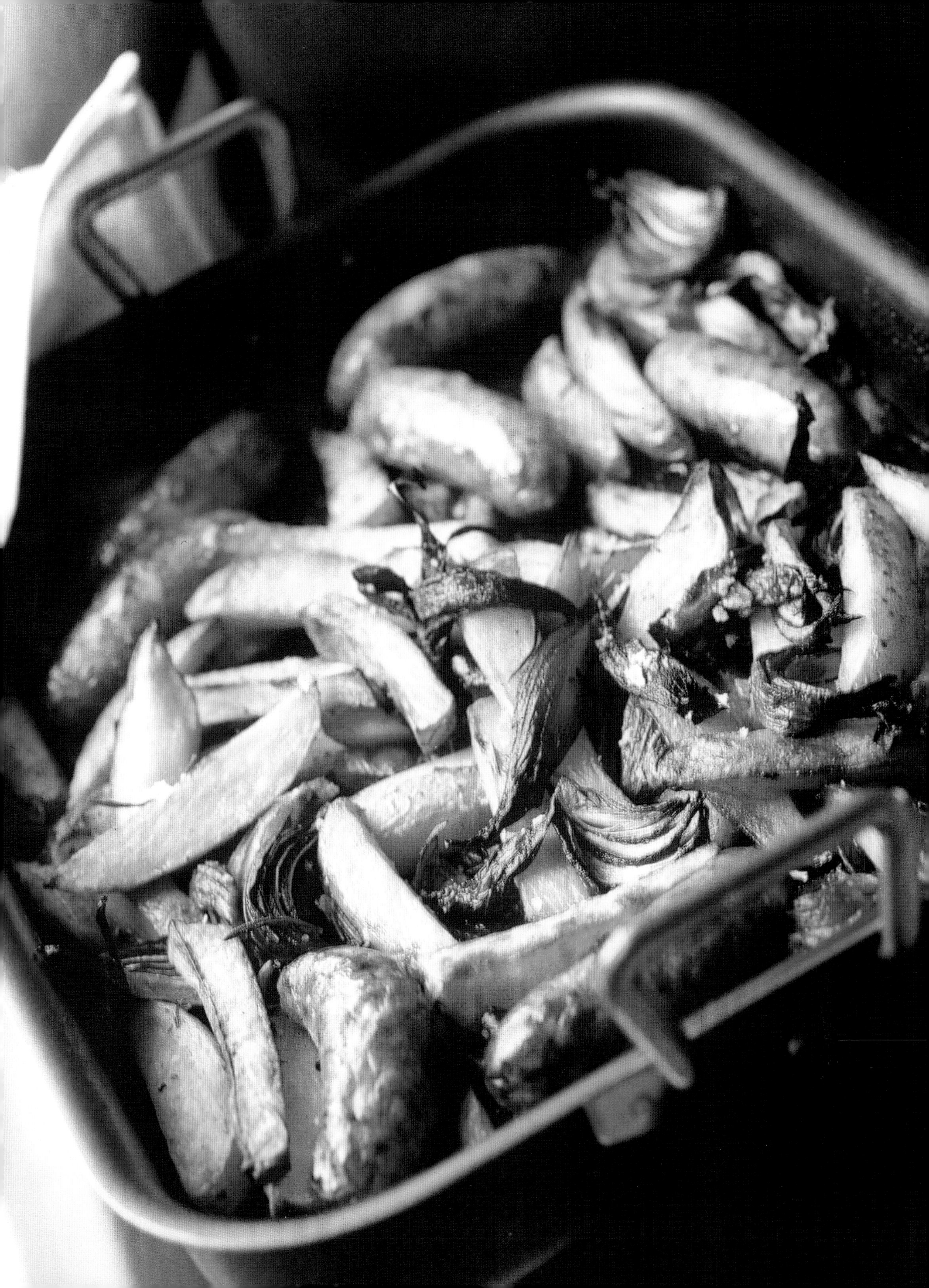

Bacon and Cabbage with Parsley Sauce

1.5kg (3lb 2oz) loin or shoulder of bacon
75g (3oz) butter
50g (2oz) plain flour
900ml (1½ pints) milk
2 level tbsp freshly chopped parsley
½ Savoy cabbage – around 900g (2lb) – finely sliced

serves 6
preparation time: 5 minutes
cooking time: 1 hour 15 minutes
per serving: 280 cals, 12g fat, 9g carbohydrate

A delicious, cheap and nutritious supper.

1 Put the bacon in a pan, cover with cold water and bring slowly to the boil. Skim off froth, cover and simmer for 20 minutes per 450g (1lb) of bacon, topping up with water from time to time. Drain, reserving the liquid.
2 Meanwhile, melt 50g (2oz) butter in a pan, add the flour and cook, stirring, for 1 minute. Reduce the heat and gradually pour in the milk, whisking constantly. Season, add the parsley, bring to the boil and simmer gently for 2–3 minutes until thickened and smooth.
3 Bring the reserved cooking water to the boil, add cabbage and cook for 8–10 minutes. Drain well, then melt remaining butter in a large pan, add the cabbage and stir-fry for 1 minute. Season well. Remove and discard the bacon rind. Serve sliced with cabbage, parsley sauce and mash.

Spicy Glazed Pork Chops

1 level tbsp curry paste
1 level tbsp mango chutney
A large pinch turmeric
1 tbsp vegetable oil
4 pork loin chops

serves 4
preparation time: 5 minutes
cooking time: 15–18 minutes
per serving: 260 cals, 15g fat, 2g carbohydrate

Don't worry if the pork chops blacken slightly while they're under the grill as this will add to the flavour of the finished dish. Serve with sautéed potatoes and grilled cherry tomatoes.

1 Put the curry paste, mango chutney, turmeric and oil in a bowl and mix well. Preheat the grill to high. Put the chops on to a grill rack, season well and brush with half the curry mixture.
2 Grill for 8–10 minutes until golden and slightly charred. Turn the chops over, season again and brush with the remaining curry mixture. Put back under the grill and cook for a further 6–8 minutes until tender and slightly charred. Serve with sautéed potatoes and grilled cherry tomatoes.

Pumpkin Mash and Sausages

500g (1lb 2oz) pumpkin, or kaobcha or harlequin squash
10 pork chipolata sausages
¼ level tsp freshly grated nutmeg

serves 4
preparation time: 10 minutes
cooking time: 40 minutes
per serving: 170 cals, 13g fat, 8g carbohydrate

Ever tasted boiled pumpkin? It often absorbs so much water that the end result is far too watery and bland. Instead, this tried and tested method of cooking pumpkin is to bake it in its skin, add a dot of butter, then scoop it straight from the shell. This gives you a super-smooth mash that tastes deliciously rich and creamy. Buy the best-quality sausages you can afford. Put the mash and sausages together and you have a delicious, hearty meal.

1 Preheat the oven to 200°C (180°C fan oven) mark 6. Put the pumpkin in a roasting tin and put in the oven to roast.
2 Cut between each sausage to separate them and add to the roasting tin after the pumpkin has been in the oven for 15 minutes. Cook for 15 minutes, then turn the sausages over so they brown evenly. Turn over the pumpkin, too, and return the tin to the oven for 30 minutes, or until the sausages are cooked and the pumpkin is tender (the skin should give slightly when touched).
3 Halve the pumpkin, then use a spoon to scoop out all the seeds and discard them. Season the roasted pumpkin flesh with salt and freshly ground black pepper, and sprinkle with the freshly grated nutmeg.
4 To serve, use a large spoon to scoop out the pumpkin flesh and divide among the plates, putting two-and-a-half pork sausages on each.

NOTE: A 500g (1lb 2oz) wedge taken from a very large pumpkin works just as well for this recipe as a whole pumpkin. Scoop out the seeds and wrap entirely in aluminium foil before putting in the oven.

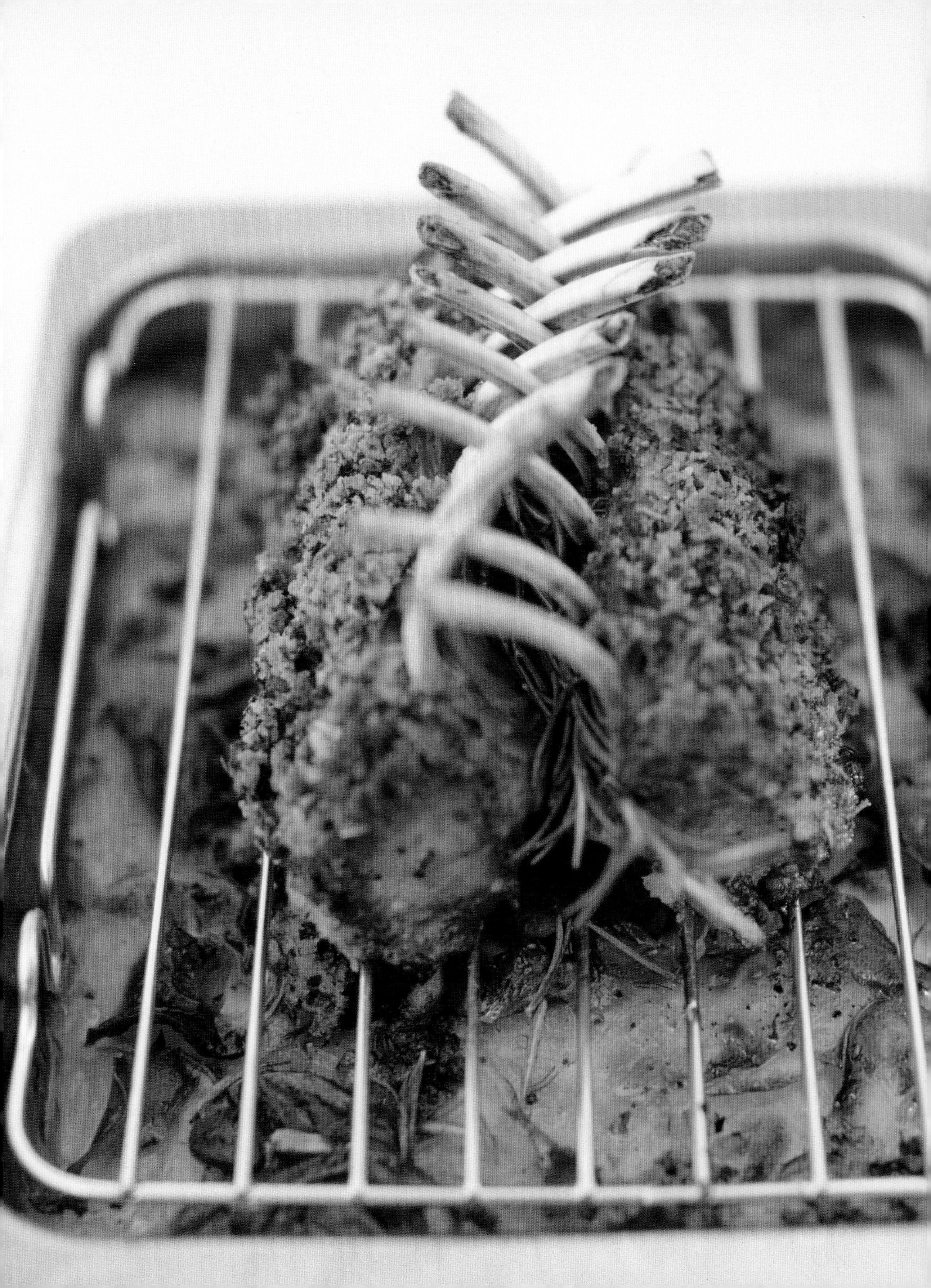

Rack of Lamb

600ml (1 pint) plain yogurt
20g (¾oz) mint, chopped
20g (¾oz) dill, chopped
3 garlic cloves, crushed
1 tbsp olive oil
2 × 8-bone French-trimmed racks of lamb
50g (2oz) breadcrumbs

serves 6
preparation time: 20 minutes, plus 24 hour marinating and 10 minutes resting
cooking time: 20–30 minutes
per serving: 320 cals, 17g fat, 12g carbohydrate

Marinating the lamb in yogurt, herbs and oil makes it meltingly tender. A crisp coating of pan-fried breadcrumbs adds colour and flavour.

1 Put the yogurt, mint, dill and garlic in a shallow bowl, season with salt and freshly ground black pepper and mix together. Put a quarter of the mixture in another bowl, cover and chill to use as a dip.
2 Add the racks of lamb to the remaining yogurt mixture and coat well. Cover and chill for at least 24 hours.
3 Preheat the oven to 200°C (180°C fan oven) mark 6. Put the lamb racks together so the bones are intersecting and put in a roasting tin. Roast for 20–30 minutes. Remove from the tin, put on a board, cover with foil and leave to rest for 10 minutes.
4 Meanwhile, heat the oil in a pan and fry the breadcrumbs until golden. Season with salt and sprinkle over the lamb racks. Serve immediately with the reserved yogurt dip.

Curried Lamb with Lentils

500g (1lb 2oz) Welsh or British lean stewing lamb on the bone, cut into eight (ask your butcher to do this)
1 level tbsp ground cumin
1 level tsp ground turmeric
2 garlic cloves, crushed
1 red chilli, deseeded and chopped
2.5cm (1in) piece root ginger, peeled and grated
2 tbsp rapeseed oil
1 onion, chopped
400g can chopped tomatoes
2 tbsp vinegar
175g (6oz) red lentils, rinsed
Traditional Mediterranean wraps
Freshly chopped coriander leaves to serve

serves 4
preparation time: 15 minutes
cooking time: 1 hour 50 minutes
per serving (not including wraps): 340 cals, 16g fat, 14g carbohydrate

Lamb is often an expensive option, but if you get the stewing variety on the bone it's really good value. This is a mild, child-friendly curry – a little meat goes a long way. Serve it with a crisp green salad and grated carrots, each dressed with a drizzle of regular malt vinegar.

1 Put the lamb into a shallow sealable container, add the spices, garlic, chilli, ginger and 1 level tsp salt. Stir well to mix, then cover and chill for 30 minutes or more.

2 Heat the rapeseed oil in a large, flameproof casserole. Add the onion and cook over a gentle heat for 5 minutes. Add the lamb and cook for 10 minutes, turning regularly, until the meat is evenly browned.

3 Add the chopped tomatoes, vinegar, 450ml (¾ pint) boiling water and the red lentils and bring to the boil. Reduce the heat, cover the casserole and simmer for 1 hour. Remove the lid and cook uncovered for 30 minutes, stirring occasionally, until the sauce is thick and the lamb is tender.

4 Remove the wraps from their plastic packaging and roll up together, then wrap in greaseproof paper or baking parchment, twisting the ends to secure. Microwave on HIGH for 1½ minutes (based on a 900W oven) until warmed through. Spread the lamb curry on the wraps. Sprinkle with fresh coriander and roll up individually to serve.

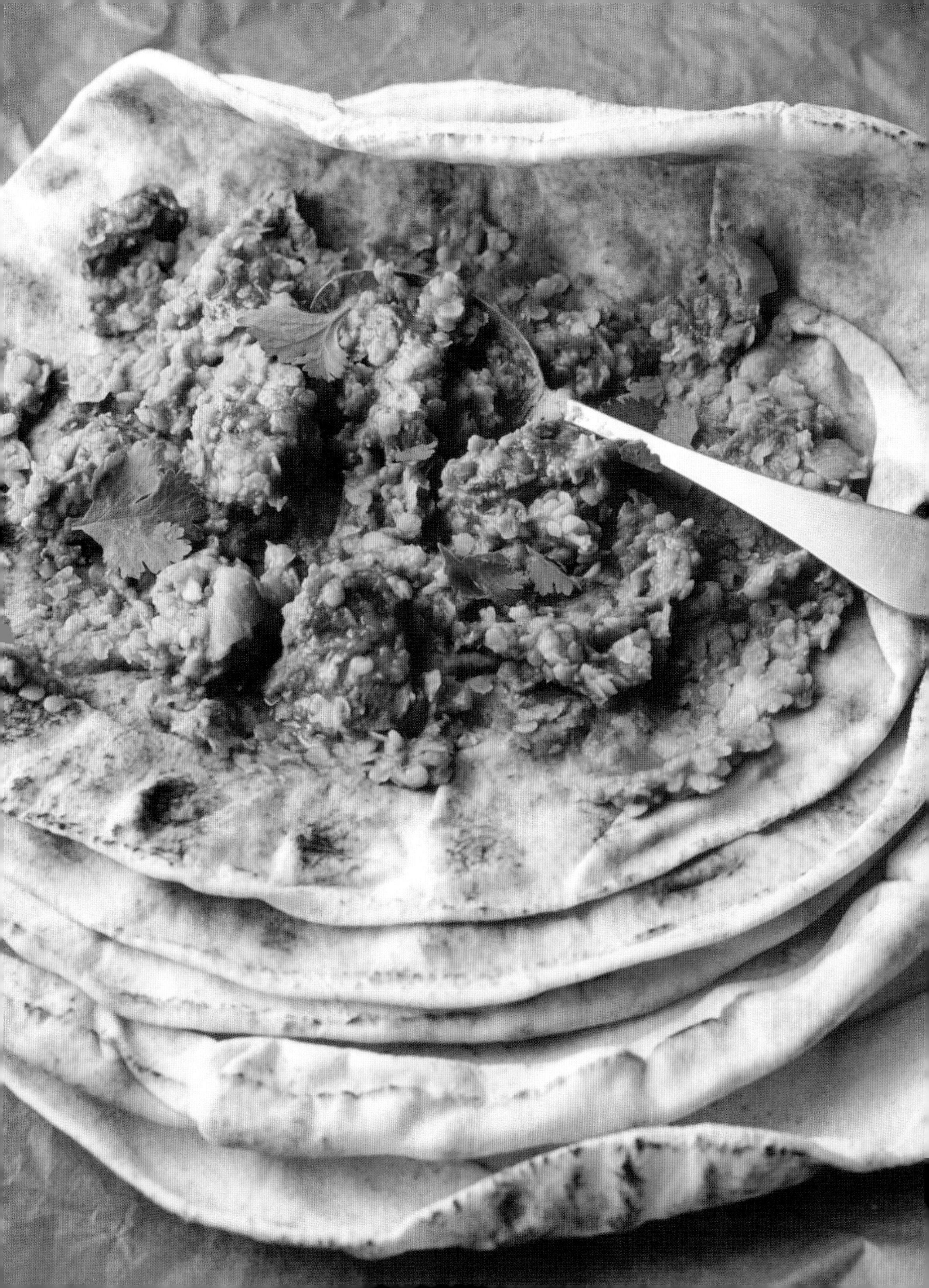

Braised Lamb Shanks with Cannellini Beans

2 tbsp olive oil
6 lamb shanks
1 large onion, peeled and chopped
3 carrots, peeled and sliced
3 celery sticks, sliced
2 garlic cloves, peeled and crushed
2 × 400g cans chopped tomatoes
100ml (4fl oz) balsamic vinegar
2 bay leaves
2 × 410g cans cannellini beans, drained and rinsed

serves 6
preparation time: 15 minutes
cooking time: about 3 hours
per serving: 430 cals, 18g fat, 28g carbohydrate

Lamb shanks are great for slow cooking – the meat becomes tender and falls off the bone. The vegetables cook down to a rich sauce, given extra flavour with balsamic vinegar.

1 Heat the olive oil in a large, flameproof casserole and brown the lamb shanks, in two batches, all over. Remove and set aside.
2 Add the onion, carrots, celery and garlic to the casserole and cook gently until softened and just beginning to colour.
3 Return the lamb to the casserole and add the chopped tomatoes and balsamic vinegar, giving the mixture a good stir. Season with salt and pepper and add the bay leaves. Bring to a simmer, cover and cook on the hob for 5 minutes.
4 Transfer to the oven and cook at 170°C (150°C fan oven) mark 3 for 1½–2 hours or until the lamb shanks are nearly tender.
5 Remove the casserole from the oven and add the cannellini beans. Cover and return to the oven for a further 30 minutes. Serve with some crusty bread – ciabatta would be perfect.

Moroccan Chicken, Squash and Chickpea Stew

1 tbsp rapeseed oil
4 boneless, skinless chicken breasts, cut into bite-sized pieces
1 onion, roughly chopped
2 garlic cloves, crushed
2.5cm (1in) piece fresh ginger, grated
2 level tbsp harissa paste
25g (1oz) plain flour
1.1 litres (2 pints) hot vegetable stock
4 tomatoes
1.4kg (3lb) butternut squash, peeled, deseeded and cut into chunks
400g can chickpeas, drained and rinsed
250g (9oz) spinach leaves
Juice of 1 lime

serves 6
preparation time: 25 minutes
cooking time: 1 hour 20 minutes–1 hour 25 minutes
per serving: 280 cals, 9g fat, 26g carbohydrate

Lean pieces of chicken, flavoured with ginger and harissa paste, in a light stew packed with chunks of squash, chickpeas and spinach.

1 Heat the oil in a large pan, add the chicken and cook over a medium heat for 5 minutes until it is browned all over, stirring occasionally. Add the onion, garlic and ginger and continue to cook for 5 minutes until softened. Add the harissa and flour and cook over a medium heat for 1–2 minutes. Add the stock, cover and bring to the boil, then reduce the heat and simmer for 45 minutes.
2 Meanwhile, score the tomatoes and plunge into a bowl of boiling water for about 30 seconds. Drain and peel off the tomato skins. Scoop the seeds into a sieve resting over a bowl (to catch any juice), then roughly chop the tomato flesh. Add to the bowl containing the juice, and put aside.
3 When the stew has simmered for 45 minutes, add the squash, chickpeas and tomatoes and their juice to the pot. Cover and bring to the boil, then simmer, stirring occasionally, for a further 20 minutes or until the squash is tender.
4 Remove any large stalks from the spinach and tear the larger leaves in half. Add to the pan with the lime juice and cook for 2–3 minutes. Season well with salt and freshly ground black pepper. Serve with crusty bread to soak up the juices.

Classic Roast Chicken

for the stuffing
40g (1½oz) butter
1 small onion, chopped
1 garlic clove, crushed
75g (3oz) white breadcrumbs
Finely grated zest and juice of 1 small lemon (reserve the lemon halves)
2 level tbsp each freshly chopped flat-leaved parsley and tarragon
1 medium egg yolk
for the chicken
1.4kg (3lb) organic chicken, skinned
2 garlic cloves
1 onion, cut into wedges
2 level tsp sea salt
2 level tsp coarse ground black pepper
4 sprigs each of fresh parsley and tarragon
2 bay leaves
50g (2oz) butter, cut into cubes

serves 5
preparation time: 30 minutes
cooking time: 1 hour 20 minutes
per 120g serving of chicken without skin: 170 calories, 5g fat, 0g carbohydrate
stuffing: 120 cals, 8g fat, 10g carbohydrate

This French-inspired garlic and herb roast is bursting with flavour and is perfect for an extra-delicious Sunday lunch.

1 Preheat the oven to 190°C (170°C fan oven) mark 5. To make the stuffing, melt the butter in a pan and fry the onion and garlic for 5-10 minutes until soft. Cool, then add the remaining ingredients, stirring in the egg yolk last. Season well.
2 Discard any string tied around the chicken, then rinse the bird in cold water. Put it on a board with the parson's nose facing upwards, then put the garlic, onion, lemon halves and half the salt, pepper and herb sprigs into the cavity.
3 Fill the neck cavity with stuffing. Turn on to its breast and pull the neck flap over the opening to cover the stuffing. Rest the wing tips across it and secure the flap with a skewer so it sits lengthways down the backbone.
4 Push a skewer through the two wings. Tie one end of a piece of string to the loop of this skewer, then turn chicken over. Pull the string up towards and around legs, then back down to the skewer in the neck flap. Pull string to tighten, then secure it.
5 Put the chicken on a rack in a roasting tin. Season, then add the remaining herbs and the bay leaves. Dot with the butter and roast for 1 hour 20 minutes (or 20 minutes per 450g/1lb, plus 20 minutes), basting halfway through, or until the juices run clear when a knife is inserted into the thigh.
6 Remove and cover with foil until ready to slice and serve.

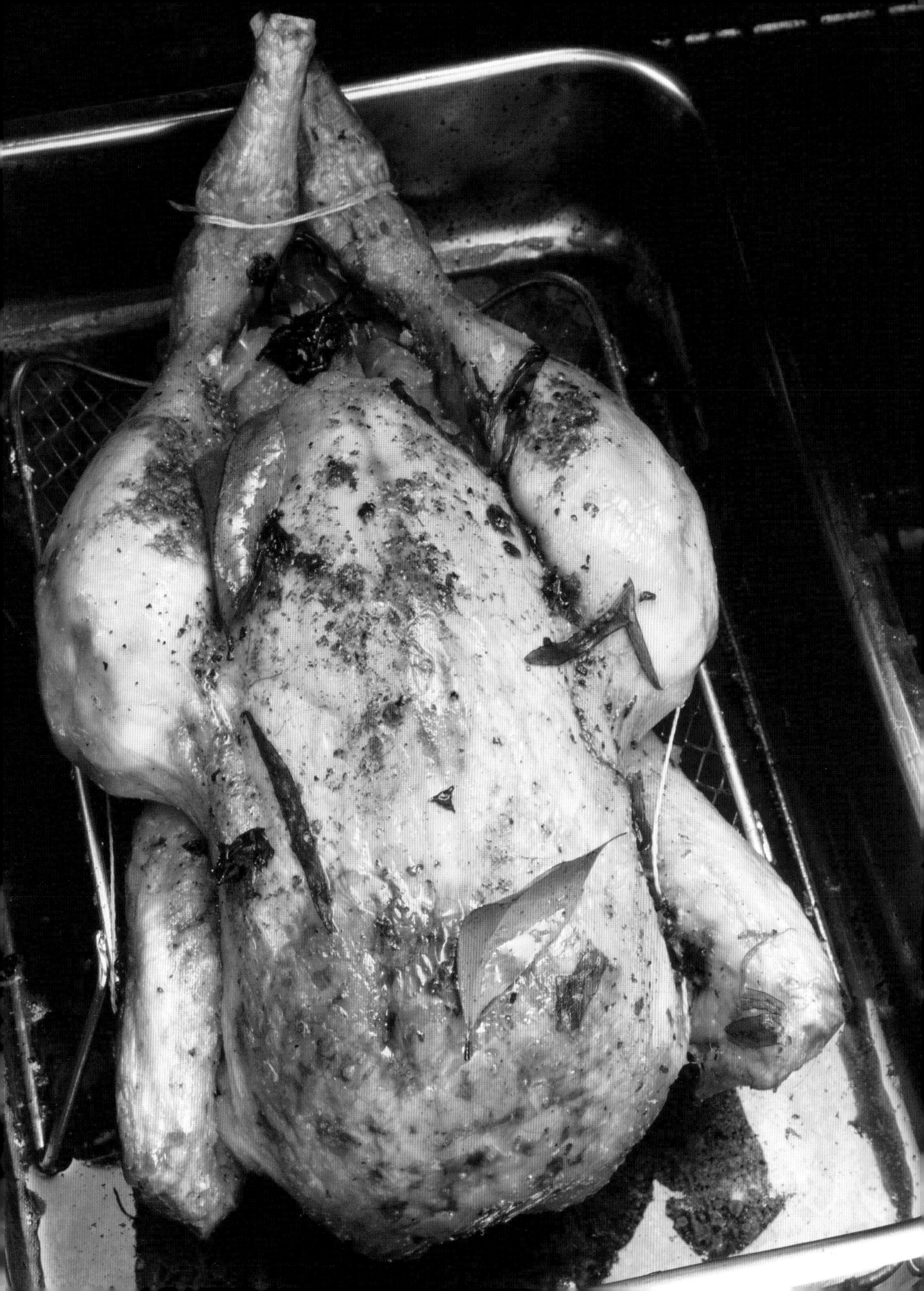

Crunchy Mangetout and Tender Chicken

2 tbsp vegetable oil
2 garlic cloves, crushed
4 skinless, boneless chicken breasts, sliced
350g carrot sticks
200g (7oz) trimmed mangetout
1 bunch spring onions, sliced
1 tbsp bottled sweet chilli sauce
250g (9oz) thick egg noodles

serves 4
preparation time: 20 minutes
cooking time: 18 minutes
per serving: 500 cals, 15g fat, 52g carbohydrate

A sweet chilli sauce adds a flavour boost to the great textures of this chicken stir-fry dish.

1 Bring a large pan of water to the boil.
2 Meanwhile, heat the oil in a wok, add the crushed garlic and stir-fry for 1–2 minutes.
3 Add the chicken and stir-fry for 5 minutes, then add the carrots and continue to cook for 5 minutes. Add the mangetout, spring onions, sweet chilli sauce and continue to cook for 5 minutes, tossing everything together.
4 Cook the noodles according to the instructions on the packet. Drain well, then add to the wok. Toss everything together, then serve in warmed bowls.

Chicken Curry with Rice

1 tbsp vegetable oil
1 medium onion, finely sliced
4 chicken breasts, skinned, boned and cut into bite-sized pieces
2 garlic cloves, crushed
2 level tbsp curry paste
400g can chopped tomatoes
450ml (3/4 pint) hot chicken stock
300ml (1/2 pint) basmati rice
250g (9oz) spinach

serves 4
preparation time: 15 minutes
cooking time: 30–35 minutes
per serving: 470 cals, 11g fat, 68g carbohydrate

This easy-cook curry could be made using chicken you may have left over from a Sunday roast.

1 Heat the oil in a large pan, add the onion and fry over a medium heat for 5 minutes until lightly golden. Add the chicken pieces and cook for 5 minutes until golden. Add garlic and curry paste, then stir-fry for 1–2 minutes.
2 Add the tomatoes and stock, then bring to the boil. Simmer, covered, for 15 minutes.
3 Meanwhile, cook the rice. Put 600ml (1 pint) water in a pan, cover and bring to the boil. Add the rice and 1 tsp salt; stir. Replace the lid, turn the heat down to its lowest setting and cook according to the timings on the pack (around 10–12 minutes). Once cooked, take the lid off and cover with a tea-towel, then replace the lid and leave for 5 minutes to absorb the steam.
4 Add the spinach to the curry and cook for 1 minute until it has just wilted. Spoon the rice on to warmed plates, add the curry and serve with mango chutney.

Turkey, Pepper and Haricot Bean Casserole

350g (12oz) dried haricot beans, soaked in cold water overnight
2 large onions, peeled
2 small carrots, peeled and cut into chunks
Bouquet garni (bay leaf, parsley and thyme)
1 tbsp olive oil
2 red chillies, deseeded and chopped
2 garlic cloves, peeled and crushed
350g (12oz) lean turkey meat, cut into bite-sized pieces
1 large red pepper, cored, deseeded and finely diced
1 large orange pepper, cored, deseeded and finely diced
2 courgettes, trimmed and finely diced
Salt and pepper
400g can chopped tomatoes
1 tbsp sun-dried tomato paste
Large handful of basil leaves

serves 6
preparation time: 20 minutes, plus overnight soaking
cooking time: 1 hour 20 minutes
per serving: 310 cals, 5g fat, 41g carbohydrate

Use lean cuts of turkey for this satisfying dish with dried beans, peppers and courgettes.

1 Drain the soaked haricot beans, put them into a large, flameproof casserole and cover with fresh water. Quarter one onion and add it to the casserole with the carrots and bouquet garni. Bring to the boil, then cover, lower the heat and simmer for 45 minutes or until the beans are tender. Drain the haricot beans, reserving 150ml (¼ pint) of the cooking liquid; discard the flavouring vegetables. Set the beans aside.
2 Finely slice the other onion. Heat the olive oil in the clean casserole, add the onion and cook gently for 5 minutes. Add the chillies and garlic and cook for 1 minute until softened.
3 Add the turkey and stir-fry for 5 minutes, then add the peppers and courgettes. Season well. Cover the casserole and cook for 5 minutes until the vegetables are slightly softened.
4 Add the tomatoes and sun-dried tomato paste, cover and bring to the boil. Add the haricot beans and reserved cooking liquid. Stir and season well with salt and pepper, then cover and simmer for 15 minutes. Stir in the basil leaves just before serving.

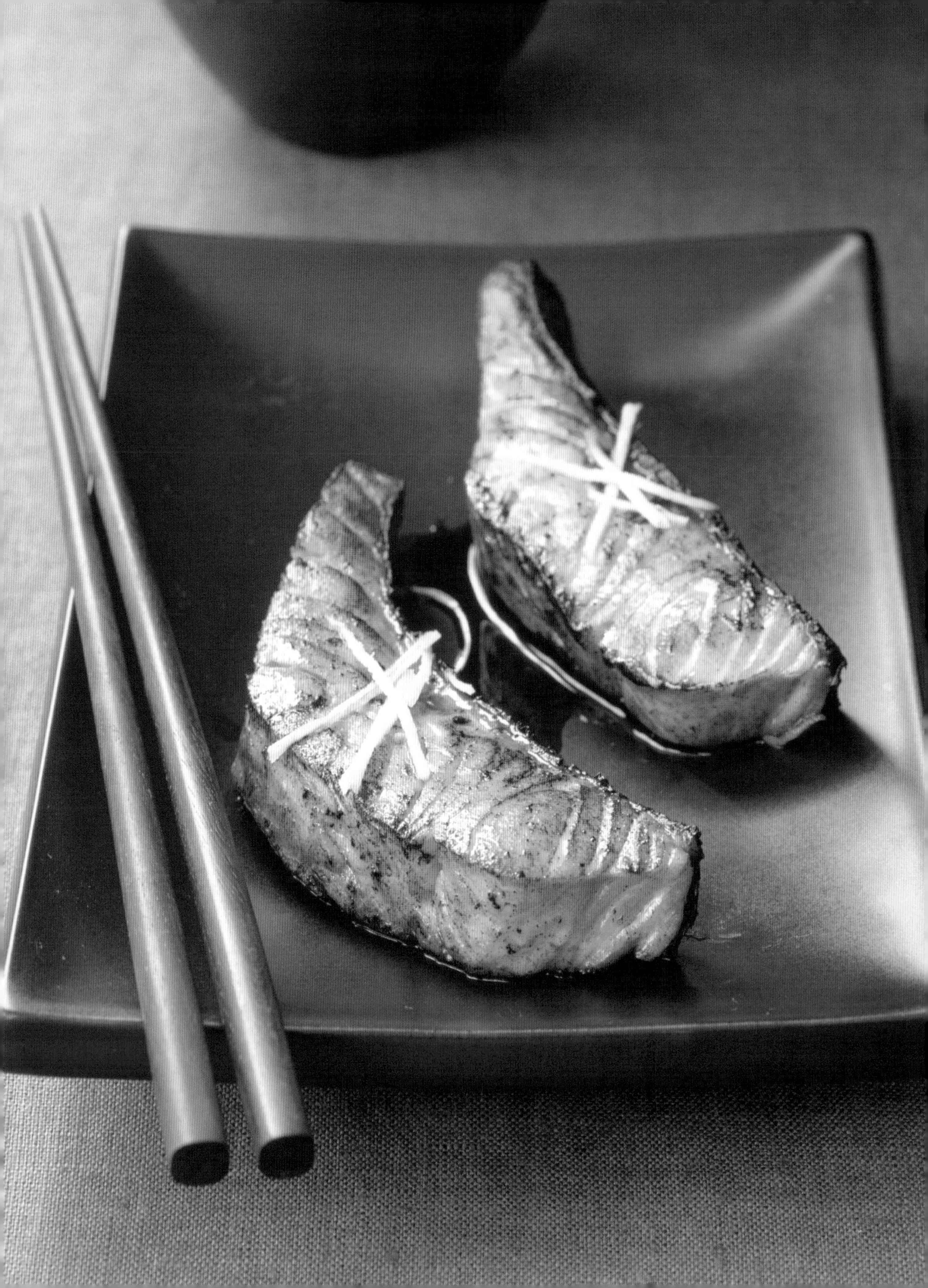

FISH

Prawn and Pak Choi Stir-fry

Thai Red Curry with Prawns

Japanese-style Salmon

Salmon Pâté with Melba Toast

Salmon and Asparagus Terrine

Oven-roast Cod with Pea Purée

Smoked Salmon Tortilla

Seafood Paella

Lemon Tuna

Ceviche of Fish with Avocado Salsa

Spicy Monkfish Stew

Lime and Chilli Swordfish

Mediterranean Fish Stew

Navarin of Cod

Pan-fried Dover Sole with Lemon

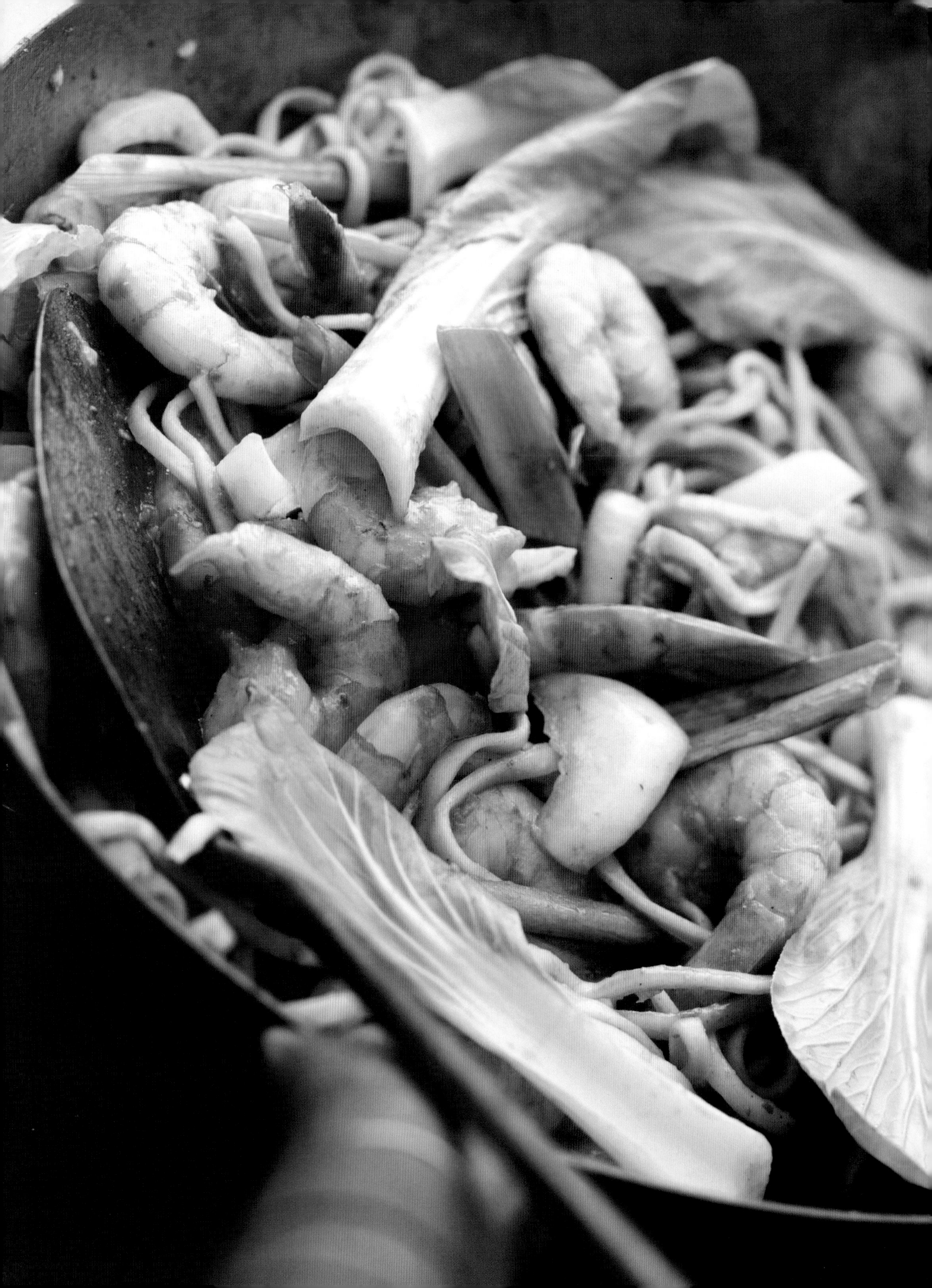

Prawn and Pak Choi Stir-fry

250g pack medium egg noodles
200g (7oz) pak choi
1 bunch of spring onions, trimmed
1 tbsp stir-fry oil or sesame oil
1 garlic clove, peeled and sliced
1 tsp grated fresh root ginger
250g (9oz) peeled raw tiger prawns, defrosted if frozen
160g jar Chinese yellow bean stir-fry sauce

serves 4
preparation time: 10 minutes
cooking time: 5 minutes plus 4 minutes standing time
per serving: 340 cals, 6g fat, 50g carbohydrate

You can't get much easier than this – it's ready and on the table in 20 minutes!

1 Put the egg noodles into a large, heatproof bowl, pour over 2 litres (3½ pints) of boiling water and leave to soak for 4 minutes. Drain and set aside. Meanwhile, cut the pak choi leaves from the white stems and set aside. Cut the white stems into thick slices. Cut each spring onion into 4 pieces. Drain the noodles and set aside.
2 Heat the oil in a wok, then stir-fry the garlic and ginger for 30 seconds. Add the spring onions and prawns and cook for 2 minutes.
3 Add the chopped white pak choi stems and the yellow bean sauce. Fill the empty sauce jar with boiling water and pour this into the wok too.
4 Add the egg noodles and continue to cook for 1 minute, tossing every now and then to heat through. Finally, add the green pak choi leaves and cook briefly until just wilted. Serve at once.

Thai Red Curry with Prawns

1 tbsp oil
1 onion, finely sliced
250g (9oz) baby aubergines, halved lengthways
1–2 tbsp red Thai curry paste
400ml can lower fat coconut milk
200ml (7fl oz) hot fish stock
1 tbsp Thai fish sauce (optional)
200g (7oz) raw tiger prawn tails, shelled
3 level tbsp roughly chopped coriander, plus extra to garnish

serves 4
preparation time: 15 minutes
cooking time: 20 minutes
per serving: 210 cals, 16g fat, 9g carbohydrate

In Thailand, this might be made with tiny pea aubergines – look out for them in Thai food shops.

1 Heat the oil in a wok or large pan and fry the onion over a medium heat until golden. Add the aubergines and fry for a further 5 minutes until pale brown.
2 Add the red Thai curry paste and stir to coat the vegetables, then continue to cook for 1 minute.
3 Add the coconut milk, stock and fish sauce, if using, then bring to the boil and simmer for 5 minutes.
4 Add the prawns and season generously with salt and freshly ground black pepper. Simmer until the prawns have turned pink – just a couple of minutes.
5 Add the coriander and stir, then transfer to large, warmed bowls and serve garnished with the extra coriander.

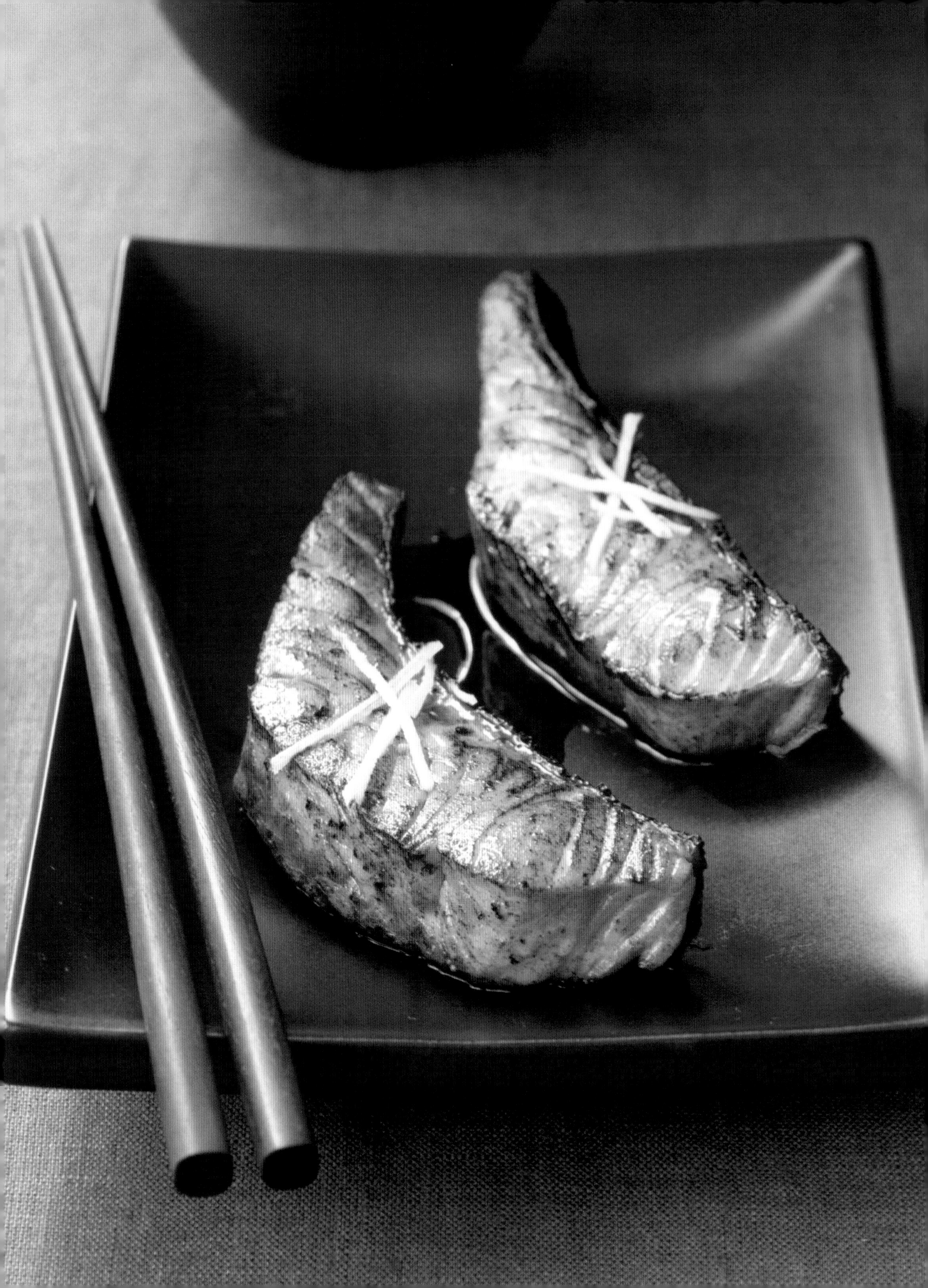

Japanese-style Salmon

550g (1 1/4lb) piece salmon fillet, with skin
4 tbsp dark soy sauce
4 tbsp mirin
2 tbsp sake
2cm (3/4in) piece fresh root ginger, peeled and cut into slivers, plus extra to garnish
1–2 tbsp oil

serves 4
preparation: 5 minutes, plus 20 minutes marinating time
cooking time: 5 minutes
per serving: 250 cals, 16g fat, 0g carbohydrate

You can easily buy ready-made teriyaki sauce, but it's good to make your own. Serve this caramelized salmon with plain boiled rice.

1 Cut the salmon fillet widthways into 4 equal pieces. Put the soy sauce, mirin, sake and ginger slivers into a shallow bowl and mix together to make teriyaki sauce.
2 Add the salmon, turn to coat and leave to marinate in a cool place for 20 minutes.
3 Heat the oil in a non-stick frying pan until very hot. Add the salmon and fry, turning occasionally, for about 5 minutes or until crisp all over. Transfer to warmed plates and top with ginger slivers to garnish. Serve with plain boiled rice.

Salmon Pâté with Melba Toast

250g (9oz) smoked salmon
3 tbsp half-fat fromage frais
1 1/2tbsp creamed horseradish
4 tbsp olive oil
1 tbsp lemon juice (around 1/2 lemon)
125g (4 1/2oz) bag baby or herb salad
for the melba toast
6 slices white bread

serves 6
preparation time: 15 minutes
per serving: 220 cals, 10g fat, 19g carbohydrate

Simple to make, and you can do it a day ahead.

1 Put the salmon in a blender and whiz to chop roughly. Add the fromage frais and horseradish and pulse briefly to combine. Put in a bowl, season with salt and ground white pepper, and chill.
2 Put the oil and lemon juice in a screw-topped jar. Season well and shake together.
3 Shape the pâté, using two dessert spoons, by scraping a spoonful of pâté from one to the other several times to form a smooth oval. Put one on each plate with a pile of salad and drizzle with dressing; serve with melba toast.
4 To make the melba toast, toast the bread, remove the crusts and cut through the middle of each slice to make two thin squares. Scrape away and discard any doughy bits. Halve each square diagonally and put on a baking sheet, untoasted side up. Grill until golden.

Salmon and Asparagus Terrine

75g (3oz) butter, plus extra for greasing
1 medium red chilli, deseeded and finely diced
1 garlic clove, chopped
½ stalk lemon grass, finely chopped
250g (9oz) asparagus spears, trimmed
250g (9oz) smoked salmon
4 level tbsp roughly chopped dill, plus extra sprigs to garnish
1kg (2¼lb) salmon fillet, skinned and boned

serves 10
preparation time: 40 minutes, plus overnight chilling
cooking time: 1 hour 5 minutes–1 hour 10 minutes
per serving: 280 cals, 19g fat, 1g carbohydrate

If you're serving a large quantity of salmon, this is a simple way to cook it. Salmon fillet is wrapped in a layer of smoked salmon and cooked in a loaf tin, which makes it very easy to slice, too.

1 Put the butter in a pan and melt over a low heat. Bring to the boil and skim off the scum until clear. Pour into a bowl and add the chilli, garlic and lemon grass. Leave to infuse.
2 Bring a large pan of cold, salted water to the boil and cook the asparagus spears for 2–3 minutes. Drain and refresh under cold water.
3 Grease and line a 900g (2lb) loaf tin with foil, then grease the foil. Line the tin with smoked salmon, reserving some for the top, and sprinkle over 1 level tbsp dill. Drizzle with a little of the infused butter and season with salt and freshly ground black pepper as you go.
4 Preheat the oven to 180°C (160°C fan oven) mark 4. Cut the salmon fillet in half to fit in the loaf tin and put one of the pieces inside. Sprinkle over 1 level tbsp dill and drizzle with a little of the infused butter. Layer up the terrine with the asparagus spears and the other salmon half, sprinkling 1 level tbsp dill and some infused butter on top of each layer and seasoning with salt and freshly ground black pepper. Finish with a layer of smoked salmon, then cover with foil.
5 Put the loaf tin in a roasting tin and half fill the roasting tin with hot water. Cook the terrine for 50–60 minutes or until a skewer inserted in the middle for 30 seconds comes out warm.
6 Leave to cool, then weight down with cans and refridgerate overnight.
7 To serve, turn out the terrine, decorate with fresh dill sprigs and cut into slices.

Oven-roast Cod with Pea Purée

2 thick cod fillets, around 200g (7oz) each
1 tbsp olive oil
375g (12oz) frozen peas
2 tbsp half fat crème fraîcbe
2 tbsp freshly chopped mint
Sea salt flakes to sprinkle
Lemon wedges to serve

serves 2
preparation time: 15 minutes
cooking time: 25–30 minutes
per serving: 360 cals, 12g fat, 18g carbohydrate

Making traditional mushy peas involves hours of soaking and boiling. This posh version – made extra creamy with a generous dollop of crème fraîche – is much quicker.

1 Dry the cod fillets with kitchen paper and season with salt and black pepper. Heat the oil in a large frying pan and cook the cod, skin-side down, until the skin is crisp. Transfer to a baking tray and cook in the oven for 15–20 minutes until the fish is tender and flaking.
2 Cook the frozen peas in boiling salted water for 8–10 minutes until very tender. Drain well and return to the pan, then add the crème fraîche and mint. Whiz to a purée with a stick blender until almost smooth.
3 Divide the pea purée between two plates. Top each with a portion of cod, then serve with a wedge of lemon to squeeze over the fish.

Smoked Salmon Tortilla

450g (1lb) potatoes, peeled
1 tbsp olive oil
1 onion, finely sliced
200g (7oz) blanched broccoli florets
75g (3oz) smoked salmon, cut into strips
4 large eggs, beaten
2 tbsp freshly chopped dill

serves 4
preparation time: 10 minutes
cooking time: 35 minutes
per serving: 260 cals, 12g fat, 24g carbohydrate

This is a tasty twist on the traditional Spanish tortilla and makes a meal in no time.

1 Cook the potatoes in a large pan of boiling, salted water for 12 minutes until just tender. Drain and set aside to cool a little.
2 Meanwhile, heat the olive oil in a 20.5cm (8in) non-stick frying pan, then fry the onion slices over a medium heat for 10 minutes until soft and golden. Remove half the mixture from the pan and set aside.
3 Slice the potatoes into rounds and put into the pan. Add the broccoli and smoked salmon, spooning over the reserved mixture as you go.
4 Preheat the grill. Stir the dill into the beaten eggs, season with salt and freshly ground black pepper and pour into the pan. Cook over a low heat for 8–10 minutes, until set underneath. Run a palette knife around the rim every couple of minutes to prevent the tortilla sticking, and make sure the tortilla doesn't catch on the bottom.
5 Pop the pan under the preheated grill and cook for 3–4 minutes until the tortilla is completely set and turning golden. Serve with a crisp green salad.

Seafood Paella

2 tbsp olive oil
2 garlic cloves, crushed
1 onion, finely chopped
2 tsp paprika
1 green pepper, deseeded and cut into strips
1 tsp saffron strands
200ml (7fl oz) passata
300g (11oz) arborio or paella rice
1 litre (1¾ pint) hot fish stock
225g (8oz) large prepared squid, sliced into rings
450g (1lb) mussels in their shells, scrubbed and beards removed
225g (8oz) raw tiger prawns, with shells on
1 lemon, cut into wedges

serves 6
preparation time: 20 minutes
cooking time: 27–30 minutes
per serving: 300 cals, 6g fat, 44g carbohydrate

There are as many different paella recipes as there are Spanish cooks. This simplified version is more typical of the southern coast of Spain.

1 Heat the oil in a large frying pan. Fry the garlic and onion for 5 minutes, add the paprika and pepper and cook for 2 minutes.
2 Stir in the saffron and passata and cook for 2 minutes. Add the rice and stir until translucent. Pour in one-third of the stock, bring to a simmer and cook for 5 minutes, until most of the liquid is absorbed. Add half of the remaining stock and cook, stirring, for 5 minutes.
3 Add the squid, mussels and prawns and stir. Pour in the remaining stock and cook for 10 minutes, stirring occasionally, until almost all the liquid is absorbed.
4 Serve garnished with lemon wedges.

Lemon Tuna

3 large lemons
2 garlic cloves, crushed
75ml (3fl oz) extra-virgin olive oil
900g (2lb) fresh tuna in one piece
3 tbsp freshly chopped flat-leaved parsley

serves 8
preparation time: 15–20 minutes, plus 30 minutes' marinating time
cooking time: 4–6 minutes
per serving: 210 cals, 11g fat, 0g carbohydrate

Fresh tuna prepared in a marinade of lemon, olive oil and garlic: simple but very tasty.

1 Soak eight bamboo skewers in a bowl of water.
2 Take two of the lemons and finely grate the zest from one and squeeze the juice from both. Mix with the garlic and olive oil and season well with freshly ground black pepper.
3 Cut the tuna in half lengthways, then cut into 8 long strips about 2cm (¾in) thick. Lay the strips in a shallow dish, pour the marinade over them, then turn the fish to coat. Cover and leave for at least 30 minutes.
4 Starting at the thinner end of each strip, roll up the tuna and thread on to a skewer, securing the ends (don't worry if any strips break – roll them up separately and thread on to the same skewer). Cut the remaining lemon into 8 wedges and push one on to each skewer. Drizzle with any remaining marinade and sprinkle with the chopped parsley.
5 Lay the skewers of tuna on the barbecue and cook for 2–3 minutes on each side.

Ceviche of Fish with Avocado Salsa

700g (1½lb) halibut fillet or Icelandic cod
Juice of 1 large orange
Juice of 6 limes
for the salsa
3 large ripe tomatoes
1 large red pepper, halved, deseeded and finely diced
2 small red chillies, halved, deseeded and finely chopped
1 red onion, diced
2 small avocados, halved, stone removed, peeled and diced
4 tbsp freshly chopped coriander
2 tbsp freshly chopped parsley

serves 4
preparation time: 10–15 minutes, plus at least 8 hour marinating time
per serving: 250 cals, 10g fat, 7g carbohydrate

Chunks of halibut or Icelandic cod are marinated in lime juice long enough for the acid to cure the fish, giving it a fresh flavour while keeping it succulent. An avocado salsa, spiked with a little chilli, complements the fish perfectly.

1 Remove any skin and bones from the fish and cut the flesh into bite-sized pieces. Put in a bowl and pour the orange and lime juices over. Turn the fish to coat completely in the juice, then cover and put in the fridge. Leave the fish to marinate for at least 8 hours or overnight.
2 To make the salsa, plunge the tomatoes into boiling water for 30 seconds, then refresh in cold water. Peel away the skin. Cut into quarters, remove the seeds, then dice. Put in a bowl.
3 Add the pepper, chillies, red onion and avocadoes to the bowl, along with the coriander and parsley. Season to taste with salt and freshly ground black pepper, then mix well.
4 To serve, drain the fish, and pile it on to six plates. Spoon the salsa over, then grind over coarse pepper.

NOTE: If you can't get hold of halibut or Icelandic cod, you can substitute any other firm-fleshed white fish such as turbot, monkfish, brill or scallops – just remember that the fish needs to be fresh.

Spicy Monkfish Stew

1 tbsp olive oil
1 onion, finely sliced
1 tbsp namjai tom yum soup paste or red Thai curry paste
450g (1lb) potatoes, cut into 2cm (¾in) chunks
400g can chopped tomatoes in rich tomato juice
600ml (1 pint) hot fish stock
450g (1lb) monkfish, cut into 2cm (¾in) chunks
200g (7oz) washed ready-to-eat baby spinach

serves 6
preparation time: 10 minutes
cooking time: 30 minutes
per serving: 160 cals, 3g fat, 18g carbohydrate

Warming, spicy fish stew makes a hearty and nutritious main course.

1 Heat the oil in a pan and fry the onion over a medium heat for 5 minutes, until golden.
2 Add the curry paste and potatoes and stir-fry for 1 minute. Add the tomatoes and hot stock, season well with salt and freshly ground black pepper and cover. Bring to the boil then simmer, partially covered, for 15 minutes or until the potatoes are just tender.
3 Add the monkfish to the pan and continue to simmer for 5–10 minutes or until the fish is cooked. Add the baby spinach leaves and stir through until wilted.
4 Spoon the fish stew into bowls and serve immediately with crusty bread.

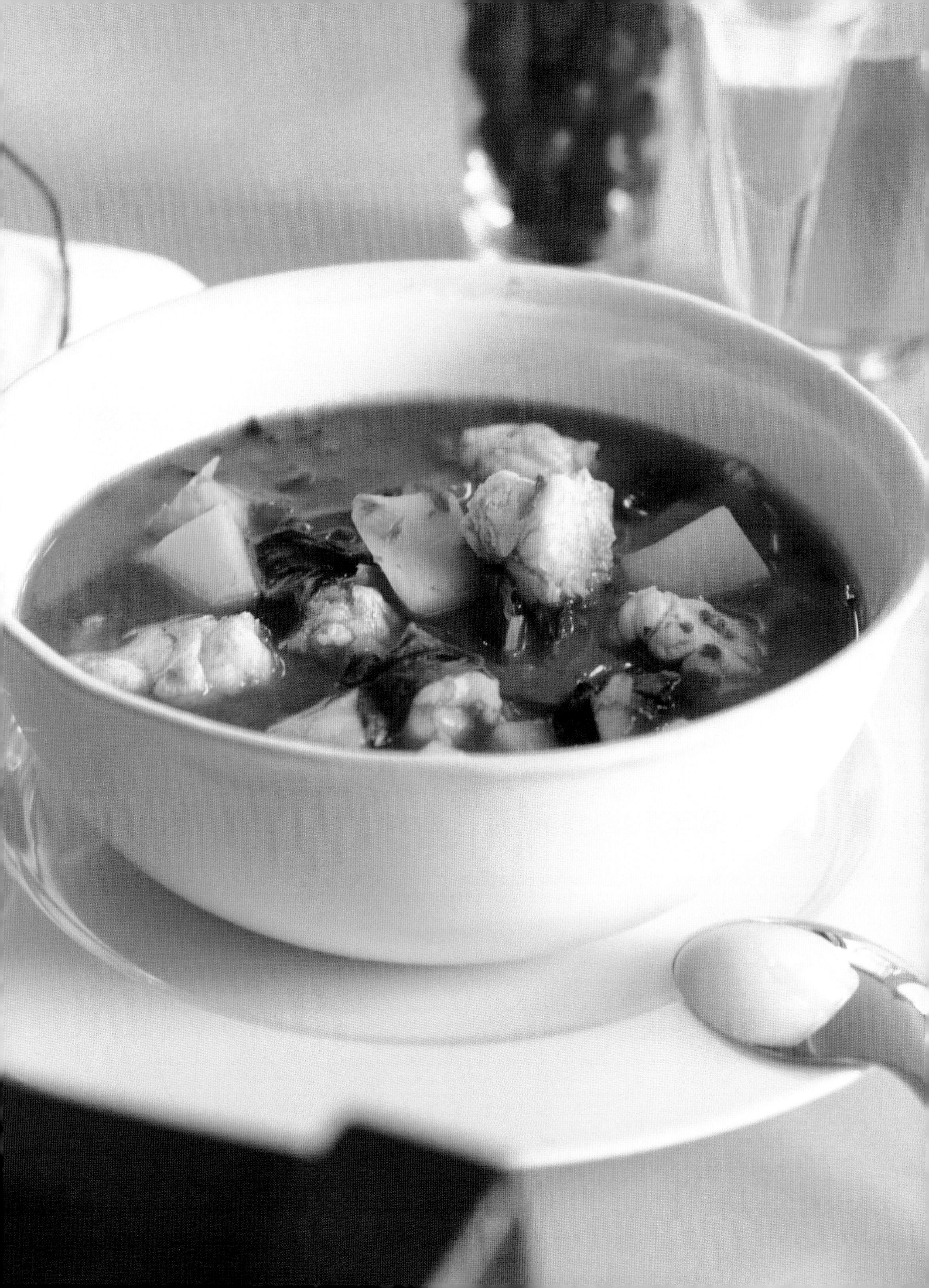

Lime and Chilli Swordfish

1 level tsp dried chilli flakes
2 tbsp olive oil
Zest and juice of lime, plus 1 whole lime, sliced, to serve
1 garlic clove, crushed
4 × 175g (6oz) swordfish steaks

serves 4
preparation time: 10 minutes, plus 30 minutes' marinating time
cooking time: 10 minutes
per serving: 190 cals, 8g fat, 0g carbohydrate

A good marinade infuses meat or fish with flavour without being overpowering, and helps to tenderize it at the same time. This recipe uses lime, dried chilli flakes and olive oil with swordfish.

1 Put the chilli flakes in a large, shallow bowl. Add the olive oil, lime zest, juice and garlic, and mix everything together. Add the swordfish steaks to the marinade and toss several times to coat completely. Leave to marinate for 30 minutes.
2 Preheat the barbecue – it's ready to use when the coals are glowing and are covered with light ash. Alternatively, preheat a griddle pan until hot.
3 Lift the swordfish out of the marinade, season well with salt and freshly ground black pepper, then cook the steaks for 2 minutes on each side. Top with slices of lime and continue to cook for 1 minute or until the fish is opaque right through.

Mediterranean Fish Stew

2 tbsp olive oil
1 small Spanish onion, peeled and finely chopped
1–2 garlic cloves, peeled and chopped
2 tsp tomato purée
pinch of powdered saffron
1 large potato, about 250g (9oz), peeled
750ml (1¼ pints) well-flavoured fish stock
½ head fennel, trimmed and thinly sliced
3 tomatoes, skinned, deseeded and sliced
225g (8oz) cod fillet, skinned
225g (8oz) monkfish fillet, skinned
4 tsp plain flour
¼ tsp cayenne pepper
Salt and pepper
125g (4½oz) peeled raw tiger prawns, deveined
1 tbsp brandy (optional)
1–2 tbsp roughly chopped flat-leafed parsley

to serve
25g (1oz) ciabatta croûtes
2 tbsp reduced calorie mayonnaise
1 teaspoon crushed garlic
2 tbsp freshly grated Parmesan cheese

serves 4
preparation time: 30 minutes
cooking time: 40 minutes
per serving: 430 cals, 21g fat, 23g carbohydrate

This stew is a heavenly combination of cod, monkfish and tiger prawns poached in a saffron broth. For a delicious lunch, serve it with crisp croûtes – toasted rounds of French bread – topped with a red pepper and garlic mayonnaise.

1 Heat the olive oil in a large pan, add the onion and cook gently for 10 minutes or until soft. Add the garlic, tomato purée and saffron, and cook for 2 minutes.
2 Cut the potato into large chunks and add to the pan with the fish stock. Bring to the boil, then lower the heat and simmer for 15 minutes. Add the fennel and tomatoes and cook for a further 5 minutes.
3 Meanwhile, cut the cod and monkfish into 4cm (1½in) chunks. Put the flour and cayenne pepper into a large plastic bag and season with salt and pepper. Add the cod and monkfish, and toss together until the pieces are completely coated. Tip them into a sieve, shaking away any excess flour.
4 Add the fish to the simmering stew and poach gently for 3 minutes until it is cooked. Don't allow it to boil or the fish will break up. Add the prawns and cook for 2 minutes or until pink.
5 If using brandy, pour it into a warm ladle, then ignite it with a taper. When the flames have died down a little, pour the brandy into the stew. Season with salt and pepper to taste and add the chopped parsley.
6 Serve the stew in warmed bowls. Mix the mayonnaise with the garlic. Spread the croûtes with the garlic mayonnaise, top with Parmesan and serve alongside for guests to add to their portion.

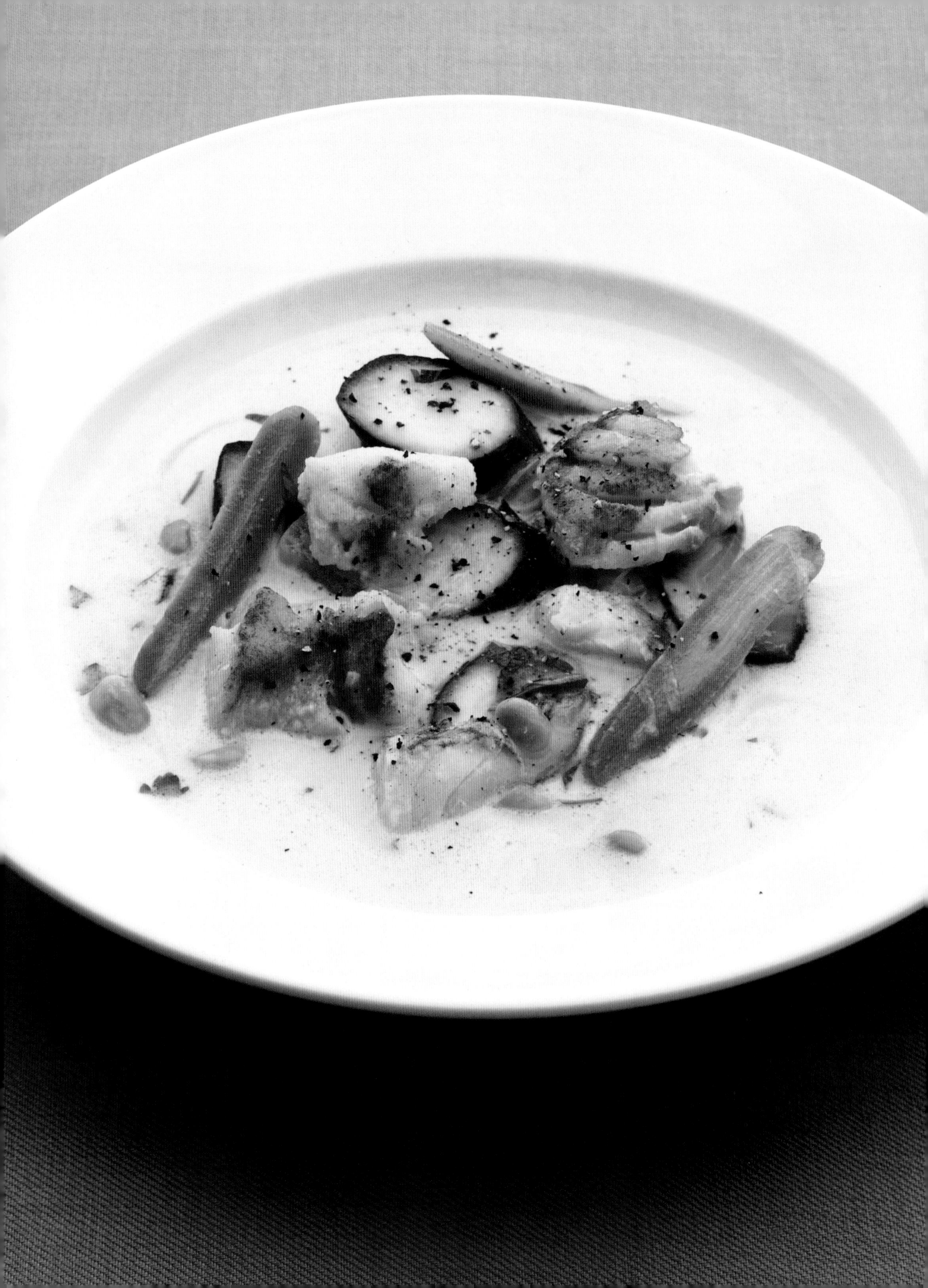

Navarin of Cod

175g (6oz) podded broad beans
25g (1oz) butter
2 tbsp sunflower oil
1 onion, peeled and sliced
225g (8oz) baby carrots, scrubbed and trimmed
225g (8oz) courgettes, trimmed and cut into 2cm (¾ inch) chunks
1 garlic clove, peeled and crushed
1.1kg (2½lb) thick chunky cod fillet, skinned
Salt and pepper
4 tbsp plain flour
150ml (¼ pint) dry white wine
300ml (½ pint) fish stock
1 tbsp lemon juice
3 tbsp double cream
2 tbsp chopped parsley

serves 6
preparation time: 15 minutes
cooking time: 25 minutes
per serving: 340 cals, 13g fat, 16g carbohydrate

A pretty, delicately-flavoured fish stew, with some early spring vegetables.

1 If the broad beans are large, blanch them in a pan of boiling water for 1–2 minutes, then drain and refresh in cold water.
2 Heat half the butter and half the oil in a large sauté pan. Add the onion, carrots, courgettes and garlic, and cook gently until softened and just beginning to brown. Remove from the pan and set aside.
3 Season the fish with salt and pepper, then dust lightly with the flour. Heat the remaining butter and oil in the pan, add the fish and brown on all sides. Remove from the pan and set aside.
4 Add the wine to the hot pan, stirring and scraping up any sediment from the bottom. Simmer for 1–2 minutes, then return the carrots, courgettes, onion, garlic and fish to the pan. Add the broad beans and stock. Bring to a simmer, then cover the pan and simmer gently for about 10 minutes or until the fish is opaque and flakes easily.
5 Stir in the lemon juice, cream and parsley. Divide among six bowls, grind some coarse black pepper on top and serve with buttered baby new potatoes.

NOTE: For a special dish, use monkfish fillet in place of cod. You'll also need to cook it for slightly longer at stage 4 – around 15 minutes.

Pan-fried Dover Sole with Lemon

2 Dover soles, about 275g (10oz) each, gutted and descaled
3 tbsp plain flour
Salt and pepper
2 tbsp vegetable oil
2 tbsp finely chopped flat-leafed parsley
Juice of ½ lemon
Lemon wedges, to serve

serves 2
preparation time: 5 minutes
cooking time: 20 minutes
per serving: 330 cals, 16g fat, 12g carbohydrate

A very quick and easy meal to cook. Simply place the fish in a pan for 5 minutes and it's done.

1 Preheat the oven to 110°C (90°C fan oven) mark ¼ and warm two dinner plates, plus another to keep the fish warm. Put the flour on a large plate and season well with salt and freshly ground black pepper. Mix in the parsley.
2 Rinse the fish under cold water, then gently pat them dry with kitchen paper. Put the flour on a large plate and season with salt and pepper. Dip the fish into the seasoned herb flour, coating both sides, and gently shaking off excess.
3 Heat 1 tbsp of the oil in a large sauté pan or frying pan, and fry one fish for 4–5 minutes on each side until golden. Transfer to a warmed plate and keep warm in a low oven. Add the remaining oil to the pan and cook the other fish in the same way.
4 Serve with lemon wedges.

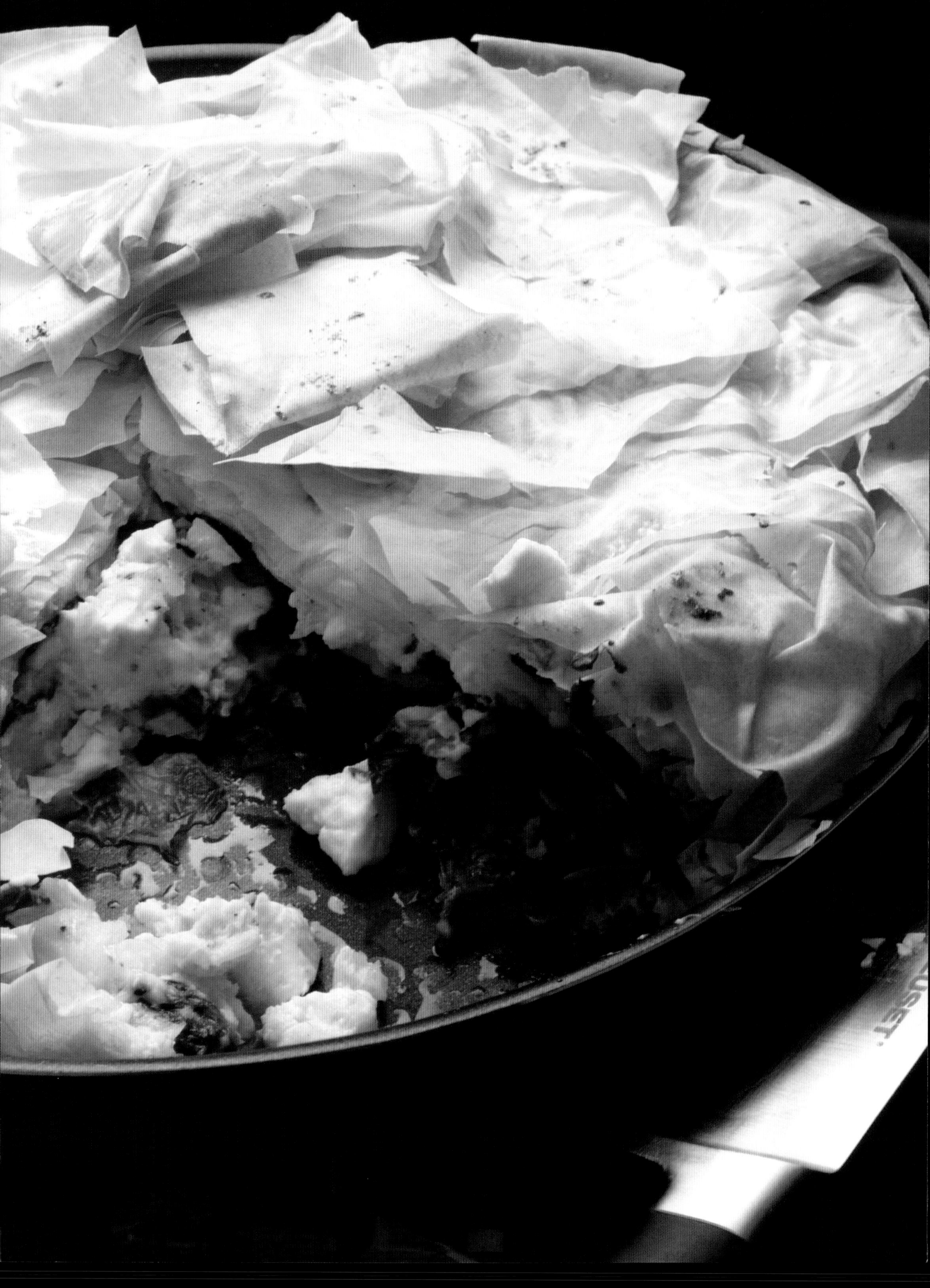

VEGETARIAN

Mint Tabbouleh

125g (4oz) bulgur wheat
150ml (½ pint) boiling water
2 tbsp extra-virgin olive oil
Juice of 1 lemon
½ diced cucumber
2 tomatoes, chopped
4 spring onions, finely chopped
2 tbsp freshly chopped mint
4 tbsp freshly chopped parsley
Seasoning

serves 4 as a side dish
preparation time: 20 minutes
per serving: 90 cals, 7g fat, 7g carbohydrate

Mint adds a fresh flavour to any savoury dish. Try this recipe, which makes enough for four people.

1 Put the bulgur wheat in a bowl, add the boiling water, cover and leave to soak for 15 minutes.
2 Put the extra-virgin olive oil in another bowl, then add the lemon juice, diced cucumber, tomatoes, spring onions and the mint and parsley.
3 Season well, then add the soaked bulgur wheat and toss together.

Florentine Fennel with White Wine

1 tbsp olive oil
750g (1lb 10oz) fennel, trimmed and sliced
150ml (½ pint) white wine
Salt and freshly ground black pepper

serves 6
preparation time: 40 minutes
per serving: 40 cals, 2g fat, 2g carbohydrate

A great side dish that will work well when served with many meals.

1 Heat the olive oil in a deep, lidded frying pan.
2 Add the fennel and white wine, then season generously with the salt and freshly ground black pepper.
3 Cover with a tight-fitting lid, bring to the boil and simmer gently for 30 minutes or until the fennel is very tender and the liquid is reduced.

Red Pepper Pesto Croûtons

1 thin French stick, sliced into 24 rounds
125g (4½oz) ready-made or homemade pesto
4 pepper pieces (from a jar of marinated peppers), each sliced into 6 strips
24 pine nuts, to garnish

makes 24
preparation time: 20 minutes, plus a little cooling
cooking time: 15–20 minutes
per serving: 80 cals, 4g fat, 9g carbohydrate

Baked bread, topped with pesto, red pepper and pine nuts. We used fresh pesto from the chiller cabinet in the supermarket.

1 Preheat the oven to 200°C (180°C fan oven) mark 6. Brush both sides of the bread with olive oil; put on a baking sheet. Bake for 15–20 minutes.
2 Spread 1 tsp pesto on each croûton, top with a pepper strip and a pine nut.

NOTE: To make pesto, roughly chop 75g (3oz) basil, 50g (2oz) Parmesan, 25g (1oz) pine nuts, ½ clove crushed garlic in a food processor. With the motor running, add 50–75ml (2–3fl oz) extra-virgin olive oil to make a paste. Season well.

Vegetable Crudités

2 small carrots
2 celery stalks
½ cucumber
1 bunch of radishes
A handful of cherry tomatoes
1 loaf of French bread
for dipping
A pot of garlic flavoured low-fat natural yogurt

serves 4
per serving: 180 calories 2g fat, 34g carbohydrate

A plate of vegetable crudités makes an easy starter and radishes are an essential ingredient. Buy radishes in bunches with their roots still attached – the leaves should look fresh, not floppy, and the bulbs should feel firm.

1 Rinse the carrots, celery stalks and cucumber, then chop into batons and arrange on a plate.
2 Trim the stalks from the radishes, rinse well, then put on the plate with the tomatoes.
3 Slice the French bread into chunks and serve the crudités with the yogurt for dipping.

Spiced Bean and Vegetable Stew

3 tbsp olive oil
2 small onions, sliced
2 garlic cloves, crushed
1 level tbsp sweet paprika
1 small dried red chilli, deseeded and finely chopped
700g (1½lb) sweet potatoes, peeled and cubed
700g (1½lb) pumpkin, peeled and cut into chunks
125g (4oz) okra, trimmed
500g passata
400g can haricot or cannellini beans, drained

serves 6
per serving: 250 calories, 8g fat, 42g carbohydrate

A satisfying stew with paprika and chilli to spice it up.

1 Heat the oil in a large heavy-based pan, add the onions and garlic and cook over a very gentle heat for 5 minutes. Stir in the paprika and chilli and cook for 2 minutes.
2 Add the sweet potatoes, pumpkin, okra, passata and 900ml (1½ pints) water. Season generously with salt and freshly ground black pepper. Cover, bring to the boil and simmer for 20 minutes until the vegetables are tender.
3 Add the beans and cook for 3 minutes to warm through.

Spiced Ratatouille with Sweet Potatoes

3 courgettes, cut into 1cm (½in) cubes
1 medium aubergine, cut into 1cm (½in) cubes
1 red onion, sliced
3 garlic cloves, sliced
1 red pepper, halved, deseeded and sliced
3 medium carrots – around 225g (8oz) cut into 1cm (½in) cubes
2 sweet potatoes – around 450g (1lb) cut into 1cm (½in) cubes
2 tbsp olive oil
½ level tsp ground allspice
2 level tsp coriander seeds
500ml carton or bottle passata

serves 6
preparation time: 25 minutes
cooking time: 60 minutes
per serving: 160 cals, 5g fat, 26g carbohydrate

This simple recipe can be made by even the most reluctant cook and makes a great meal for when you have friends round for an informal supper.

1 Preheat the oven to 200°C (180°C fan oven) mark 6. Take two large roasting tins and put the courgettes, aubergine, red onion, garlic and pepper into one and the carrots and sweet potatoes into the other. Drizzle both lots of vegetables with olive oil and sprinkle with allspice and coriander seeds. Toss well.
2 Roast the vegetables for 20 minutes, then turn and continue to roast for 20 minutes until tender and slightly charred. To prepare ahead, cool, put in an airtight container and chill until needed.
3 To serve, preheat the oven to 200°C (180°C fan oven) mark 6. Put the roasted vegetables in a roasting tin, add the passata and toss well. Season generously and cook for 20 minutes.
4 To serve in a neat shape, put a 7.5cm (3 in) plain cutter on a serving plate, spoon in the ratatouille and lift up the cutter.

Spinach-baked Eggs with Mushrooms

2 tbsp olive oil
125g (4oz) chestnut mushrooms, quartered
225g bag washed baby leaf spinach
salt and pepper
2 large eggs

serves 2
preparation: 5 minutes
cooking time: 13 minutes
per serving: 250 cals, 21g fat, 2g carbohydrate

The ultimate comfort food: an egg cooked until the white has set while the yolk is still soft and runny. Fresh spinach and mushrooms add a touch of luxury to this simple dish.

1 Heat the olive oil in a large frying pan, add the mushrooms and stir-fry for 30 seconds, then add the spinach and stir-fry until wilted. Season with a little salt and pepper and divide between two 600ml (1 pint) ovenproof dishes.
2 Carefully break an egg into the centre of each dish. Season.
3 Bake at 200°C (180°C fan oven) mark 6 for about 12 minutes or until the eggs are just set. (Remember that they will continue to cook a little once they're out of the oven.) Serve immediately.

Goat's Cheese and Walnut Salad

1 large radicchio
2 bunches of watercress, trimmed
1 red onion, peeled and finely sliced
100g pack mild goat's cheese
100g walnut pieces
dressing
2 tbsp freshly squeezed orange juice
2 tbsp red wine vinegar
2 tbsp unsweetened fresh orange juice
2 tbsp olive oil
Large pinch of golden caster sugar
Salt and pepper

serves 6
preparation: 10 minutes
per serving: 180 cals, 16g fat, 5g carbohydrate

A classic French salad. Use a mild, soft goat's cheese which will crumble easily over the leaves.

1 Tear the radicchio leaves into bite-sized pieces and put into a large salad bowl with the watercress and red onion.
2 To make the dressing, put the orange juice, wine vinegar, olive oil, sugar, salt and pepper into a screw-topped jar and shake well to combine.
3 Pour the dressing over the salad and toss well. Crumble the goat's cheese on top and sprinkle with the walnuts. Serve with slices of multi-grain French bread as a starter, or light lunch.

NOTE: Mild Welsh goat's cheese is an ideal choice for this salad.

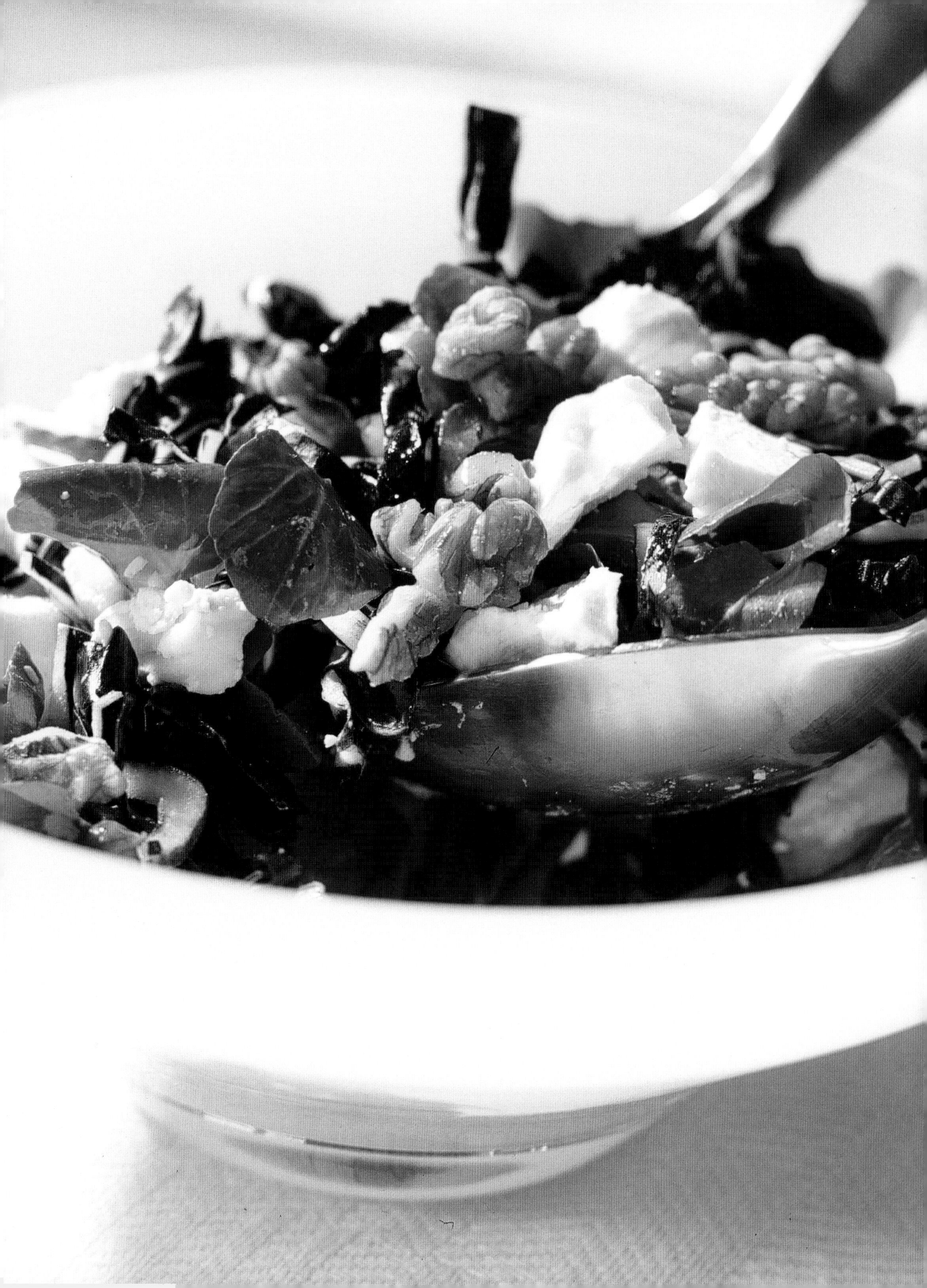

Cheese and Onion Potato Soufflé

700g (1½lb) floury potatoes, peeled and
cut into chunks
1 onion, peeled and finely chopped
Salt and pepper
15g (½oz) butter, plus extra to grease
15g (½oz) plain flour
300ml (½ pint) milk
100g (3½oz) Parmesan cheese, freshly grated, plus extra to finish
3 medium eggs, separated
1 tbsp Dijon mustard

serves 8
preparation: 30 minutes
cooking time: about 1 hour
per serving: 200 cals, 9g fat, 19g carbohydrate

This is a great dish made from eggs and a Parmesan cheese sauce folder together with mashed potato. It's important to season the sauce and the mash well first to ensure everything is well flavoured.

1 Put the potatoes and onion into a pan of cold salted water. Cover, bring to the boil and simmer, partly covered, for 15–20 minutes until tender. Drain, tip back into the pan and put over a low heat to dry a little. Mash well, seasoning with salt and pepper to taste. Cool a little.
2 Meanwhile, make the sauce. Melt the butter in a pan, stir in the flour and cook for 1 minute. Gradually stir in the milk and cook, stirring, over a low heat for 5–10 minutes until thickened. Stir in the grated Parmesan and season well with salt and pepper. Set aside to cool a little.
3 Add the cheese sauce, egg yolks and mustard to the mashed potato and mix everything together. Check the seasoning.
4 In a clean, grease-free bowl, whisk the egg whites until they stand in stiff peaks, then gently fold into the potato mixture.
5 Spoon the mixture into a buttered 1.2 litre (2 pint) soufflé dish. Stand on a baking sheet and grate over a little more Parmesan. Bake at 200°C (180°C fan oven) mark 6 for 40 minutes until risen and golden. Serve immediately.

Tomato, Basil and Olive Salad

700g (1½lb) on-the-vine tomatoes, sliced
2 × 200g tub Pomodorino (baby plum) tomatoes, halved lengthways
20 basil leaves, roughly torn
340g jar queen green olives in brine, drained
3 tbsp balsamic vinegar
2 tbsp extra-virgin olive oil

serves 12
preparation time: 15 minutes
per serving: 60 cals, 5g fat, 3g carbohydrate

A refreshing and tasty salad that makes the most of summer flavours.

1 Layer all the tomatoes in a glass bowl with basil and olives, seasoning as you go with salt and black pepper.
2 To make the dressing, put the balsamic vinegar and olive oil in a screw-top jar. Seal and shake well, then pour over the salad. Chill for up to 4 hours until needed.

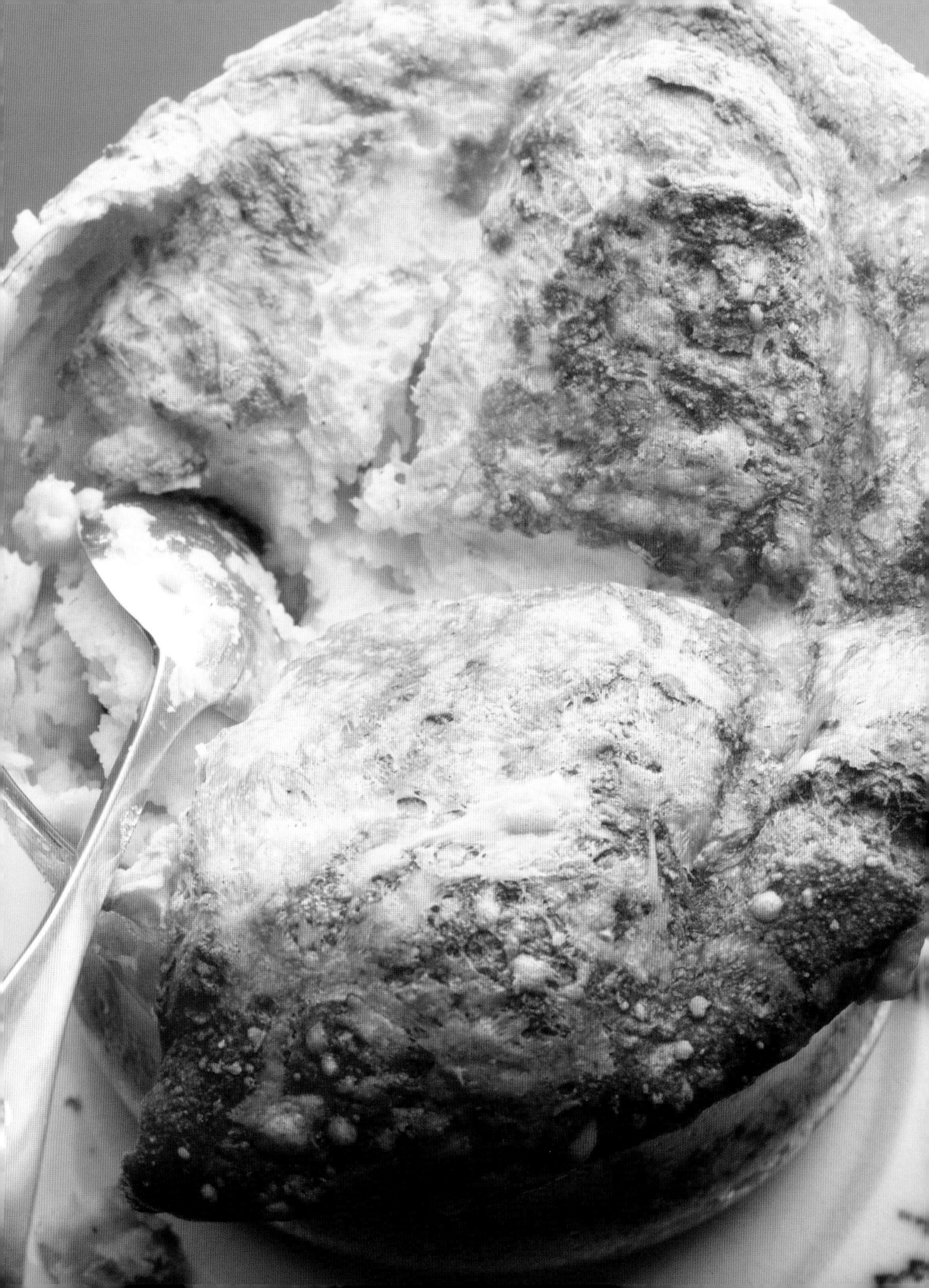

Sweet Pepper Stew

4 tbsp olive oil
2 garlic cloves, crushed
4 red peppers, sliced
3 orange peppers, sliced
1 green pepper, sliced
2 tbsp capers in brine, rinsed
18 black olives
1 tbsp freshly chopped flat-leafed parsley

serves 6–8
preparation time: 15 minutes
cooking time: 40 minutes
per serving: 120–90 cals, 10–8g fat, 7–6g carbohydrate

Known as pepperonata, this traditional dish is made by cooking peppers slowly over a low heat to bring out their full sweetness. It's best made two or three days ahead to allow all the flavours to marinate, and you can serve it warm or cold.

1 Heat the oil in a very large pan, add the garlic and stir-fry over a medium heat for 1 minute. Add the peppers, season well with salt and freshly ground black pepper and stir well to toss in the oil.
2 Cover the pan with a lid and continue to cook over a low heat for 40 minutes, stirring occasionally to prevent sticking.
3 Add capers, olives and parsley and stir. Serve immediately or cool, chill and enjoy a couple of days later with crusty bread.

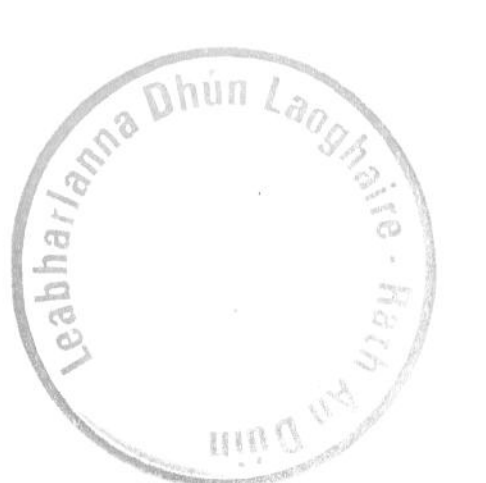
Leabharlanna Dhún Laoghaire

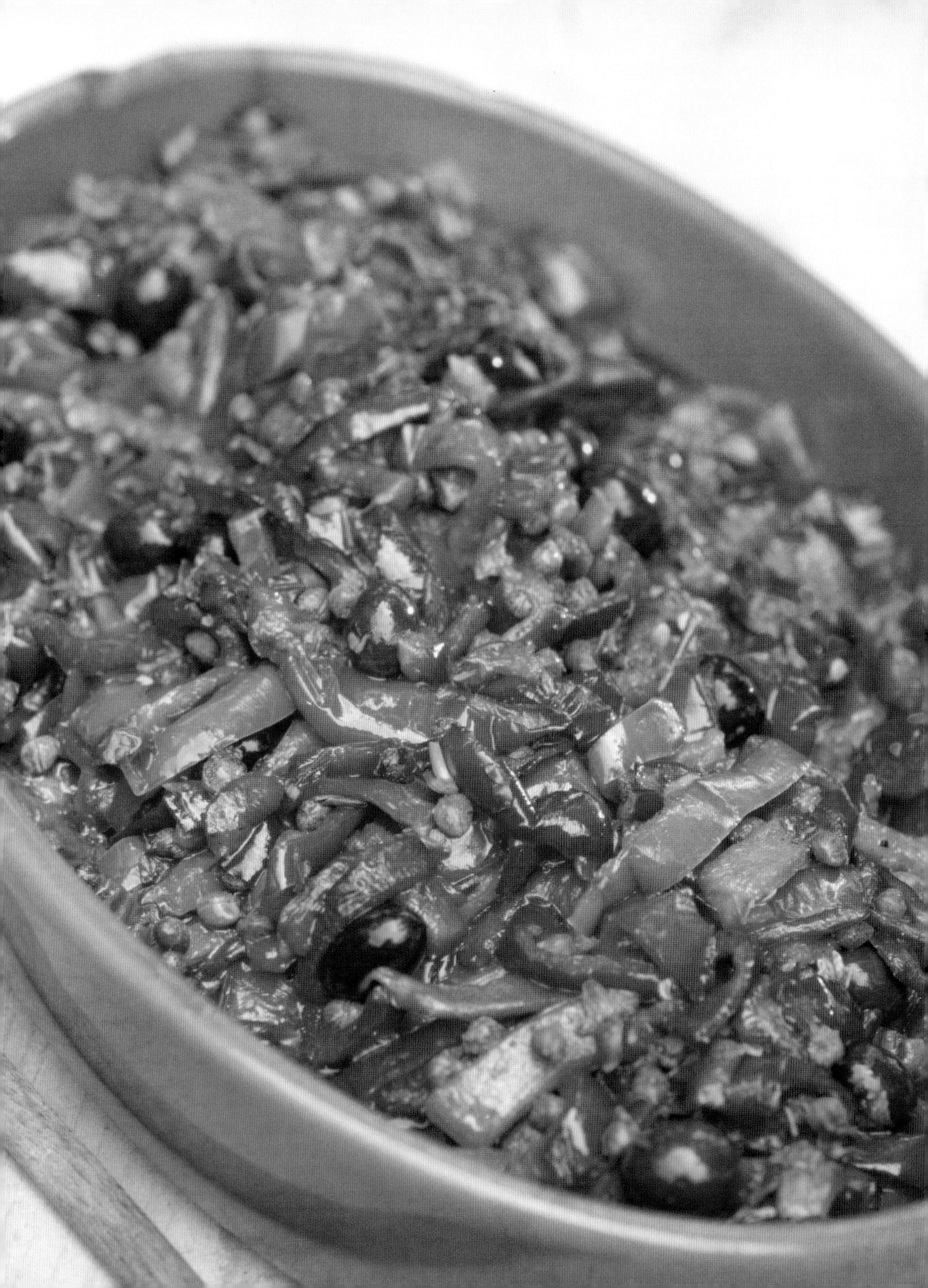

Chickpea Curry

2 tbsp vegetable oil
2 onions, finely sliced
2 garlic cloves, crushed
1 level tbsp ground coriander
1 level tsp mild chilli powder
1 tbsp black mustard seeds
2 level tbsp tamarind paste
2 level tbsp sun-dried tomato paste
750g (1lb 11oz) new potatoes in their skins, quartered
400g can chopped tomatoes
1 litre (1¾ pint) hot vegetable stock
250g (9oz) green beans, trimmed
2 × 400g cans chickpeas, drained
2 level tsp garam masala

serves 6
preparation time: 20 minutes
cooking time: 40–45 minutes
per serving: 220 cals, 7g fat, 35g carbohydrate

Ground coriander, mustard seeds and garam masala give this curry a good depth of flavour. Serve with warm naan bread and a spoonful of natural yogurt.

1 Heat the oil in a pan and fry the onions for 10–15 minutes until golden. Add the garlic, coriander, chilli, mustard seeds, tamarind paste and sun-dried tomato paste. Cook for 1–2 minutes until the aroma from the spices is released.
2 Add the potatoes and toss in the spices for 1–2 minutes. Add the chopped tomatoes and stock and season with salt and freshly ground black pepper. Cover and bring to the boil. Simmer, half covered, for 20 minutes until the potatoes are just cooked.
3 Add the beans and chickpeas, and continue to cook for 5 minutes until the beans are tender and the chickpeas are warmed through. Stir in the garam masala and serve.

Split Pea Roti

125g (4oz) yellow split peas, soaked in cold water overnight
½ level tsp turmeric
1 level tsp ground cumin
1 garlic clove, finely sliced
1½ level tsp salt
225g (8oz) plain flour, sifted
1½ level tsp baking powder
1 tbsp vegetable oil
125–150ml (¼ pint) skimmed milk
A little oil for frying

serves 4
preparation time: 25 minutes, plus 30 minutes resting
cooking time: 40 minutes
per serving: 170 cals, 3g fat, 32g carbohydrate

Healthy and great-tasting, accompany these fried rotis of split peas with a green salad.

1 Put the peas, turmeric, cumin, garlic and 1 level tsp salt into a small pan. Add 200ml (7fl oz) cold water, bring to the boil, cover with a lid and simmer for 30 minutes, or until the peas are soft, adding a little more water if necessary. Set aside to cool.
2 Put the flour, baking powder and the remaining salt into a large bowl. Make a well in the centre, add the oil and gradually mix in enough milk to form a soft dough. Transfer to a lightly floured surface and knead. Cover with a damp tea-towel and leave to rest for 30 minutes.
3 Whiz the cooled peas in a processor until smooth, adding 1tbsp water.
4 Divide the dough into eight portions. On a lightly floured surface, roll each piece out to make 20.5cm (8 in) rounds. Spread four with the pea mixture, then top with the other rounds and press to seal the edges.
5 Heat a heavy-based frying pan, brush each roti with a little oil and fry in batches for 1–2 minutes on each side or until lightly brown.
6 Serve cold or cover and heat in a 900W microwave on HIGH for 1 minute 30 seconds.

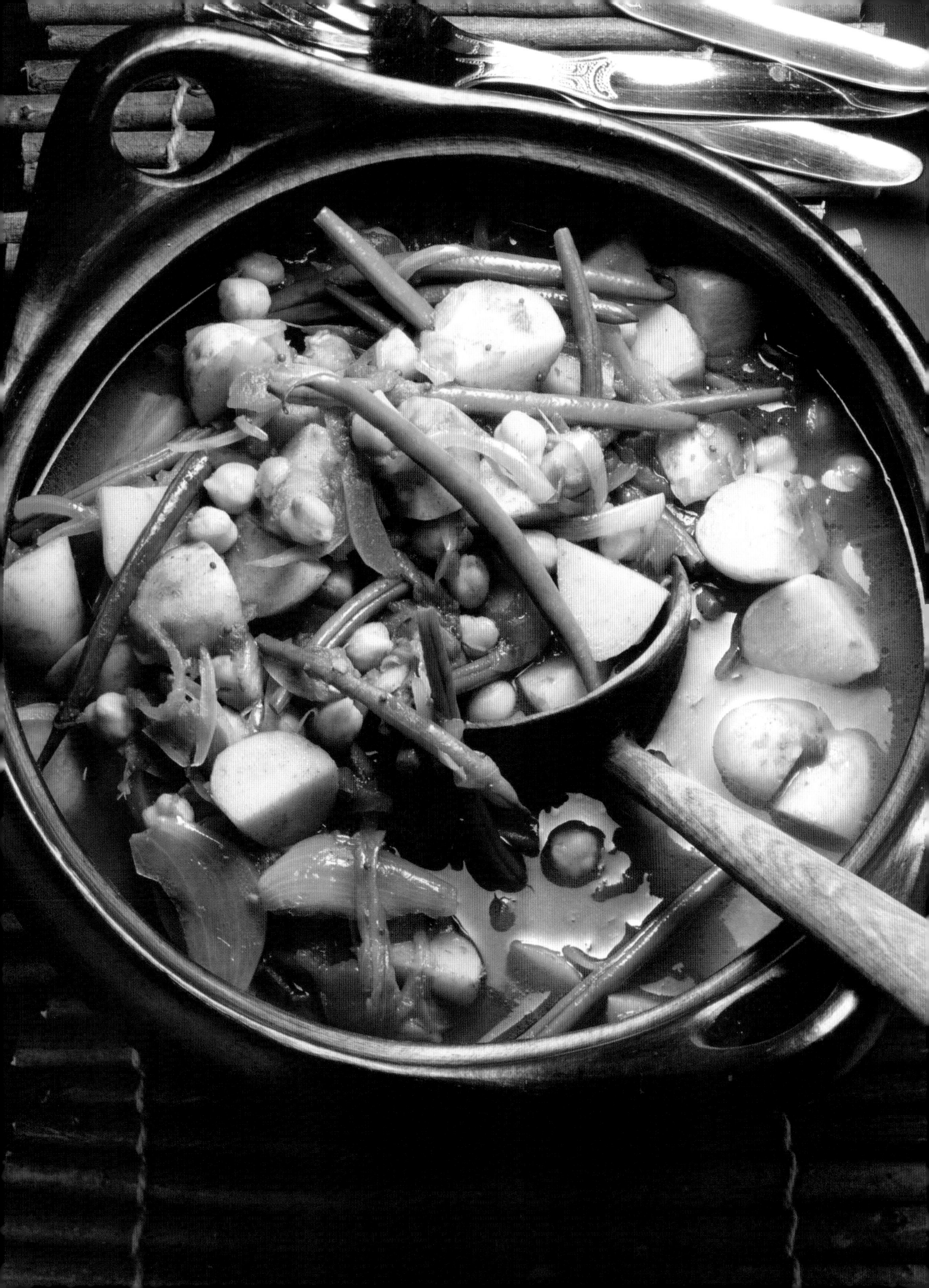

Classic Saag Aloo

900g (2lb) potatoes
2 tbsp oil
1 onion, finely sliced
2 garlic cloves, finely chopped
1 level tbsp black mustard seeds
2 level tsp turmeric
4 handfuls baby spinach leaves

serves 4
preparation time: 15 minutes
cooking time: 55 minutes
per serving: 250 cals, 7g fat, 43g carbohydrate

A traditional Indian dish of onions cooked with chunks of potato, spinach and spices. Serve it with tandoori chicken and a cucumber and yogurt dip.

1 Cut the potatoes into 4cm (1½in) chunks. Heat the oil in a pan and fry the onions over a medium heat for 10 minutes until golden, taking care not to burn them.
2 Add the garlic, mustard seeds and turmeric and cook for a further 1 minute.
3 Add the potatoes, 1 level tsp salt and 150ml (¼ pint) water and cover. Bring to the boil, then lower the heat and cook gently for 35–40 minutes or until tender.
4 Add the spinach and cook until the leaves just wilt. Serve immediately.

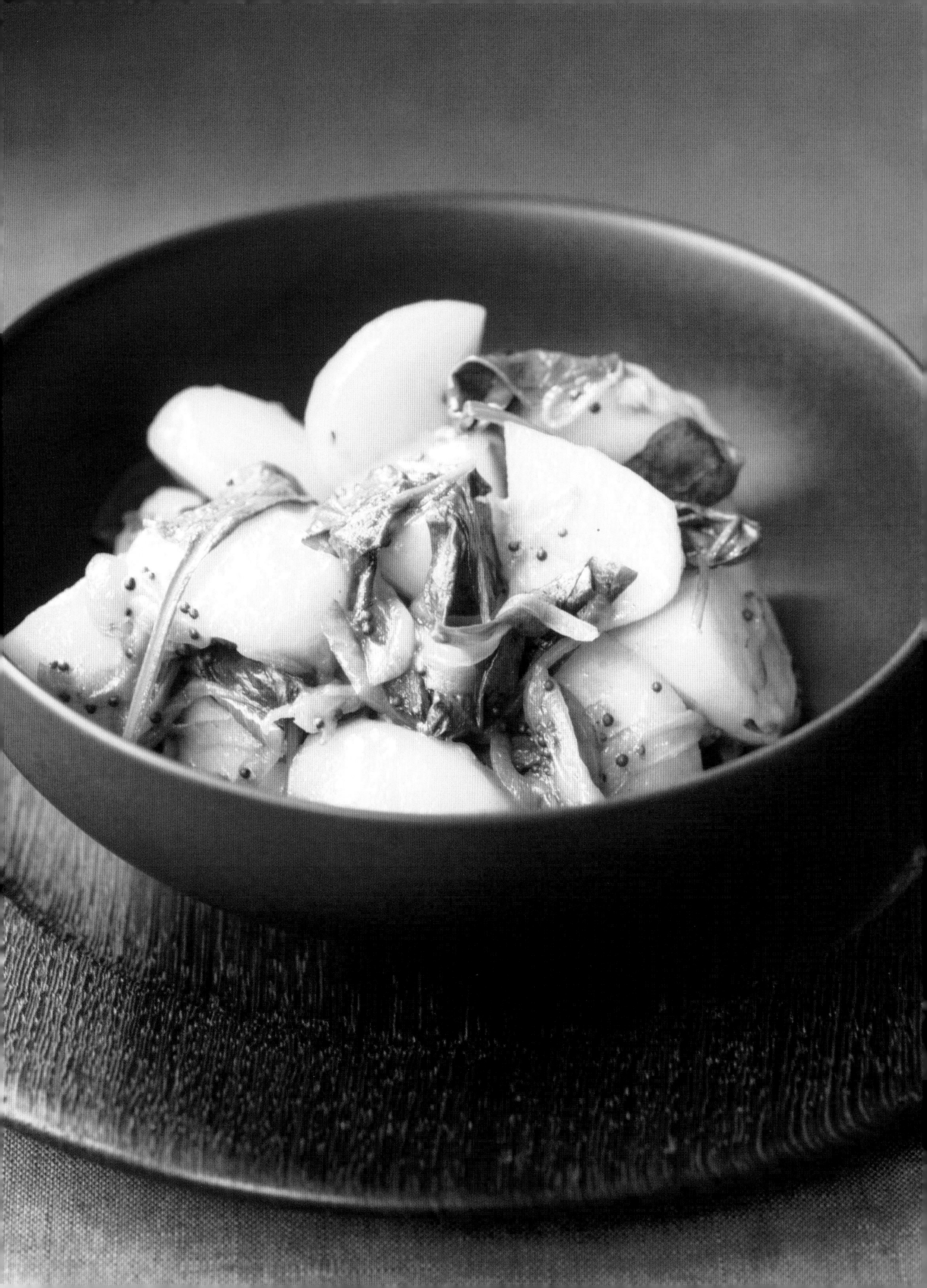

Vegetable Curry

2 tbsp rapeseed oil
1 onion, finely sliced
4 garlic cloves, crushed
2.5cm (1in) piece root ginger, grated
3 level tbsp medium curry powder
6 fresh curry leaves
150g (5oz) potato, peeled and cut into 1cm (½in) cubes
125g (4oz) aubergine, cut into 2cm (1in) long sticks, 5mm (¼in) wide
150g (5oz) carrots, peeled and cut into 5 mm (¼in) dice
900ml (1½ pints) vegetable stock
A pinch of saffron
150g (5oz) green beans, trimmed
75g (3oz) frozen peas
3 tbsp chopped fresh coriander

serves 4
preparation time: 20 minutes
cooking time: 30 minutes
per serving: 170 cals, 9g fat, 19g carbohydrate

To make ahead, cool immediately after adding the peas and beans and chill. To reheat, put in a pan, cover and bring to the boil, then simmer for 10–15 minutes.

1 Heat the oil in a large heavy-based pan. Add the onion and fry over a gentle heat for 5–10 minutes until golden. Add the garlic, ginger, curry powder and curry leaves and fry for a further 1 minute.
2 Add the potatoes and aubergines to the pan and fry, stirring, for 2 minutes. Add the carrots, stock, saffron, 1 tsp salt and plenty of black pepper. Cover and cook for 10 minutes until the vegetables are almost tender.
3 Add the beans and peas to the pan and cook for a further 4 minutes.
4 Transfer to a serving dish, sprinkle with coriander.

Roasted Ratatouille with Herb Dumplings

1 large red onion, peeled and sliced
2 garlic cloves, peeled and crushed
2 courgettes, trimmed and sliced
1 medium aubergine, trimmed and diced
2 red peppers, halved, deseeded and cut into chunky slices
4 tbsp olive oil
Salt and pepper
2 × 400g cans chopped tomatoes
dumplings
125g (4oz) self-raising flour, plus extra to dust
50g (2oz) vegetable suet
1 tbsp chopped parsley
1 tsp thyme leaves
1 litre (1¾ pints) hot vegetable stock

serves 4
preparation time: 25 minutes
cooking time: 1–1¾ hours
per serving: 410 cals, 25g fat, 41g carbohydrate

Red peppers, courgettes, aubergines and onions are roasted first in the oven to soften and sweeten, then cooked with tomatoes to turn this classic vegetarian stew into something extra special. Dumplings are an easy way to enrich the recipe, and add a flavour boost. Even better, the dish can be prepared ahead, so it's perfect for easy entertaining.

1 Put the onion, garlic, courgettes, aubergine and peppers into a roasting tin and mix them all together. Drizzle with olive oil and season well with salt and pepper. Roast at 200°C (180°C fan oven) mark 6 for 40–50 minutes.
2 Add the tomatoes and stir thoroughly. Return to the oven for 15–20 minutes.
3 Meanwhile, make the herb dumplings. Put the flour, vegetable suet, parsley and thyme leaves into a bowl and season well with salt and pepper. Add 6–7 tbsp cold water and mix everything together with a knife. Dust your hands with a little flour and shape the mixture into 4 dumplings.
4 Bring the stock to the boil in a medium pan, then reduce the heat. Add the dumplings and poach gently for 5 minutes, turning once with a slotted spoon.
5 Divide the ratatouille among four ovenproof serving dishes and put a dumpling into each dish. Stand the dishes on a baking tray and put into the oven for 10 minutes until the dumplings are lightly browned. Allow to stand for 3 minutes before serving.

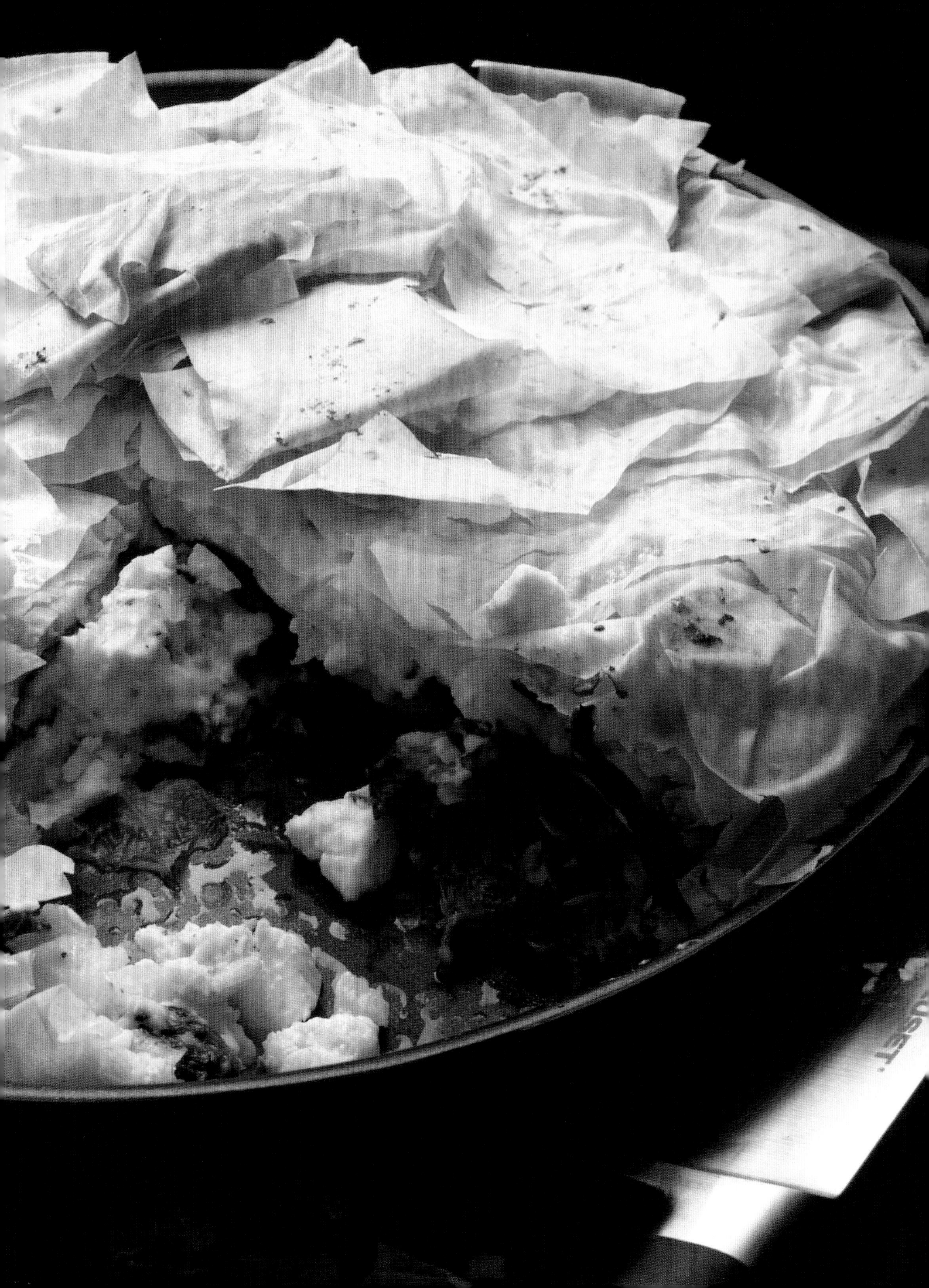

Spinach and Feta Cheese Pie

1kg (2lb 3½oz) waxy potatoes, such as Desirée, unpeeled
2 tsp rapeseed oil
1 onion, finely chopped
1 garlic clove, crushed
1 level tbsp cumin seeds
500g bag baby leaf spinach, washed and ready to use
1½ × 200g packs feta cheese, crumbled
2 medium eggs, beaten
Spray oil, for greasing
200g pack filo pastry
40g (2oz) butter, melted

serves 10
preparation time: 25 minutes
cooking time: about 1 hour
per serving: 280 cals, 13g fat, 31g carbohydrate

A filling of spinach, feta, potato and cumin, wrapped in crisp filo pastry, makes a wonderfully wholesome pie. There's enough for ten people, so if you don't eat it all, you can enjoy it cold the next day or warm it up in the oven. Serve with a crisp green salad.

1 Put the potatoes in a pan of salted water. Cover and bring to the boil, then cook for 15–20 minutes until tender. Drain and cool, then peel and slice.
2 Meanwhile, heat the oil in a large pan and cook the onion for 10 minutes until soft. Add the garlic and cumin and cook for 1–2 minutes. Add the spinach, cover and cook until the spinach has just wilted – about 1–2 minutes. Tip into a bowl and allow to cool a little.
3 Add the potatoes, feta cheese and eggs, and season with salt and freshly ground black pepper. Mix together.
4 Preheat the oven to 200°C (180°C fan oven) mark 6. Lightly spray a 28cm (11in) round, loose-based tart tin that is 3cm (1¼in) deep with spray oil. Unroll the pastry and use scissors to cut the sheets lengthways into three. Work with one-third of the strips at a time and cover the rest with clingfilm to keep moist. Lay a strip on the tin, starting from the middle so that half covers the tin and half hangs over the edge. Brush with butter, then lay another strip next to it, slightly overlapping, and brush again. Repeat, working quickly, until the tin is covered and the pastry is used up. Cover and set aside any broken pieces of pastry.
5 Tip the filling into the middle and flatten out to the edges. Quickly fold in the overhanging pastry, making sure the filling is covered and using the broken pieces to fill any gaps. Drizzle with the remaining melted butter, then bake in the oven for 45 minutes until golden and cooked through.

NOTE: To save time, cook the onion with the oil in the microwave on HIGH for 5 minutes (based on a 900W oven) until soft. Add the garlic and cumin and cook for 1 minute. You can also cook the spinach in its bag in the microwave – pierce the bag once and cook on medium for 3 minutes.

To reheat the pie, preheat the oven to 200°C (180°C fan oven) mark 6 and put the pie on a baking sheet. Cook in the oven for 15–20 minutes until hot right through.

Sweet Potato Mash

2 medium potatoes (around 400 g/14oz) such as King Edward, cut into chunks
900g (2lb) sweet potatoes, cut into chunks
50g (2oz) butter

serves 6
preparation time: 10 minutes
cooking time: 20 minutes
per serving: 240 cals, 7g fat, 42g carbohydrate

The mix of regular and sweet potatoes gives this mash a rounded, earthy taste.

1 Put both types of potato in a large pan of cold, salted water. Cover and bring to the boil, then simmer, half covered, for 15–20 minutes until tender.
2 Drain well, add the butter and season well with salt and freshly ground black pepper. Mash until smooth and serve with the roast lamb.

Asparagus with Lemon Dressing

Finely grated zest of ½ lemon
2 tbsp lemon juice
2 tbsp extra-virgin olive oil
250g (9oz) fine-stemmed asparagus, ends trimmed

serves 5
preparation time: 15 minutes
cooking time: 5 minutes
per serving: 60 cals, 6g fat, 1g carbohydrate

Tender, fine English asparagus stems signify summer. Serve them with a light citrus and olive oil dressing as an easy, healthy alternative to hollandaise sauce or butter. Delicious warm or cold.

1 Put the lemon zest into a screw-topped jar, add the lemon juice and olive oil, then shake to mix.
2 Half fill a frying pan with boiling salted water. Add the asparagus, then cover and simmer for 5 minutes or until just tender.
3 Remove the asparagus with a large draining spoon. If serving the asparagus cold, plunge it into a large bowl of iced water – this will help keep its bright green colour – then drain.
4 To serve, arrange the asparagus in a concentric pattern in a large, shallow bowl, with tips outwards and ends overlapping in the centre. Season generously with salt and freshly ground black pepper, and drizzle with the dressing.

Braised Red Cabbage

½ medium red cabbage, (approximately 500 g), shredded
1 red onion, peeled and finely chopped
1 Bramley apple, peeled, cored and chopped
1 cinnamon stick
A pinch of ground cloves
½ tsp freshly grated nutmeg
2 tbsp each red wine vinegar and red wine
Juice of 1 orange

serves 8
preparation time: 10 minutes
cooking time: 1 hour
per serving: 30 cals, trace fat, 7g carbohydrate

This is a great accompaniment to roasts because it doesn't contain oil or butter, so it cuts through the richness of the meat. We've added cinnamon and cloves, both of which work well with apple.

1 Put all the ingredients into a large pan, season with salt and freshly ground black pepper, and stir to mix well.
2 Put the pan, covered, on to a low heat and cook gently for about 1 hour, stirring the cabbage from time to time to prevent it burning on the bottom.
3 When the cabbage is tender, remove the pan from the heat and discard the cinnamon stick. Cool, put into a bowl, cover, and chill the cabbage overnight. To reheat, put it into a pan, add 2 tbsp cold water and cover with a tight-fitting lid. Heat gently for 15 minutes, stirring frequently.

Roasted New Potatoes with Herby Cheese

750g (1lb 10oz) baby new potatoes
50g (2oz) soft herb cheese
1 level tbsp finely chopped chives

makes 24–30
preparation time: 10 minutes, plus 5–10 minutes' cooling time
cooking time: 35 minutes
per serving: 40 cals, 2g fat, 5g carbohydrate

Roasted baby potatoes filled with garlicky cheese – the most moreish of canapés.

1 Preheat the oven to 200°C (180°C fan oven) mark 6. Put the potatoes in a pan of cold salted water, cover and bring to the boil. Cook for 10 minutes until tender. Drain well.
2 Tip the potatoes into a roasting tin, add a little olive oil and season with salt and freshly ground black pepper. Toss well. Roast for 25 minutes, shaking the tin occasionally, then cool for 5–10 minutes.
3 Cut a cross in the top of each potato. Squeeze them a little and spoon ⅓ tsp soft cheese into each. Sprinkle with chives. Serve warm or at room temperature.

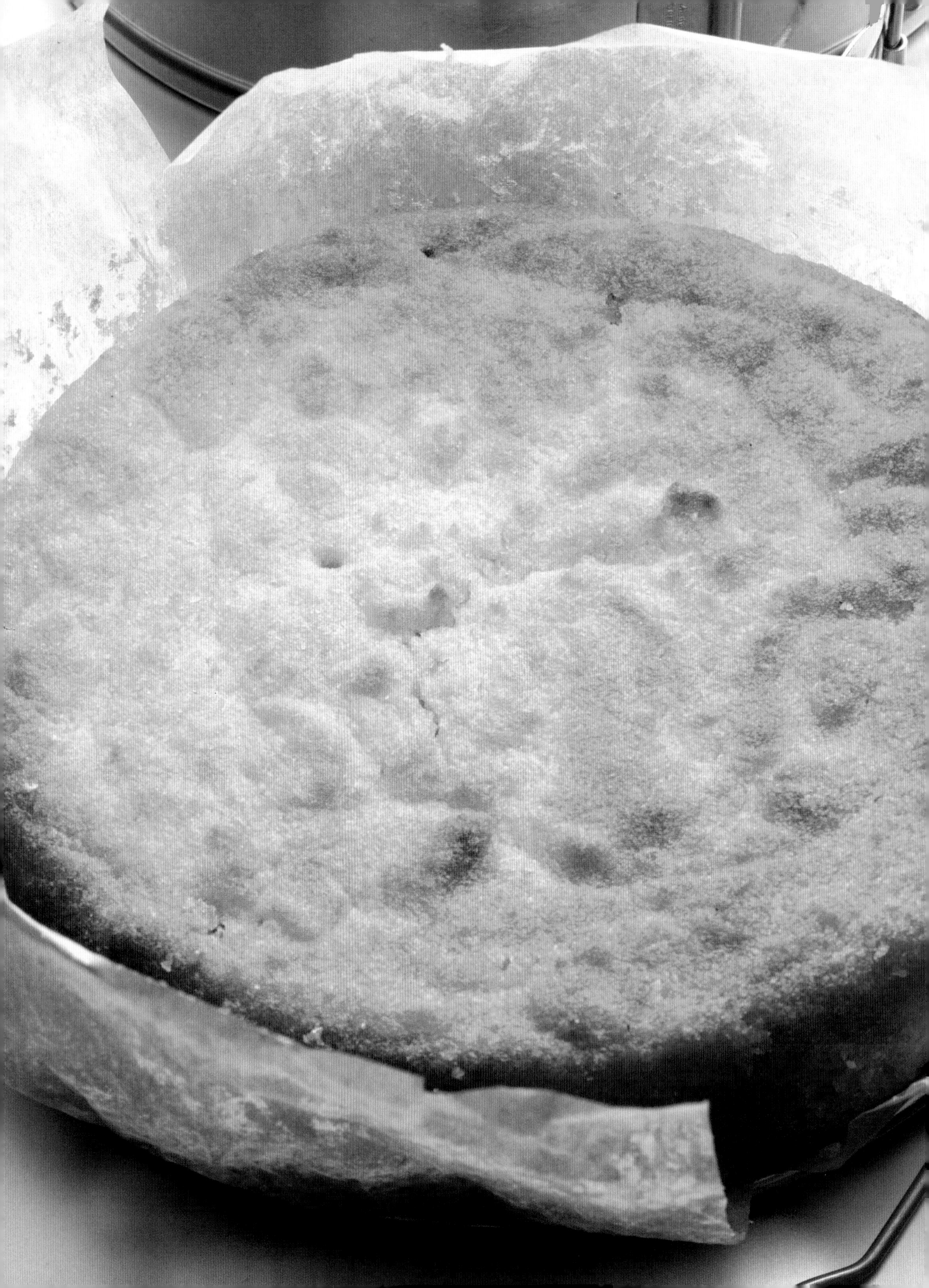

DESSERTS

Mango and Lime Mousse

Mango and Lime Swiss Roll

Rhubarb Crumble

Spiced Pears in Mulled Wine Syrup

Chocolate Cinnamon Sorbet

Orange Sorbet

Orange Meringue Terrine

Lemon Sorbet

Fresh Vanilla Custard

Sparkling Fruit Jellies

Christmas Pudding Parfait

Baked Apples

Grand Marnier Oranges and Passion Fruit

Passion Fruits and Strawberry Terrine

Moist Carrot Cake

Strawberry Sorbet

Almond and Orange Torte

Rice Pudding

Blueberry Muffins

Fruity Rice Pudding

Instant Banana Ice Cream

Mango and Lime Mousse

2 very ripe mangoes, peeled
100ml (4fl oz) whipping cream
finely grated zest and juice of 2 limes
10g (¼oz) sachet powdered gelatine
3 large eggs, plus 2 large yolks
50g (2oz) golden caster sugar
to decorate
Finely pared lime zest, shredded

serves 6
preparation time: 20 minutes, plus chilling
per serving: 180 cals, 10g fat, 17g carbohydrate

A light mousse of exotic mango and zesty lime makes a perfect ending to a summer meal.

1 Cut the mango flesh away from the stone and whiz in a blender or food processor to give 300ml (½ pint) purée. Lightly whip the cream in a bowl and set aside.
2 Put 3 tbsp lime juice into a small, heatproof bowl, then sprinkle with the powdered gelatine and leave to soak for 10 minutes.
3 In a large bowl, whisk the eggs, egg yolks and sugar together, using an electric beater, until thick and mousse-like; this will take about 4–5 minutes. Gently fold in the mango purée, cream and grated lime zest.
4 Set the bowl of softened gelatine over a pan of boiling water and leave until dissolved, then carefully fold into the mango mixture, making sure everything is evenly combined. Pour the mousse into glasses and chill for 2–3 hours until set. Decorate each mousse with shredded lime zest.

Mango and Lime Swiss Roll

A little vegetable oil to grease
125g (4½oz) golden caster sugar, plus extra to dust and dredge
125g (4½oz) plain flour, plus extra to dust
3 medium eggs
Zest of 1 lime
for the filling
200g (7oz) low-fat crème fraîche, drained of any liquid
1 tsp lime juice
1 medium mango, peeled, stoned and sliced

serves 8
preparation time: 20 minutes
cooking time: 15–17 minutes
per serving: 150 cals, 4g fat, 28g carbohydrate

This version of the classic Swiss roll is laced with lime zest for a zingy flavour and filled with low-fat crème fraîche and succulent mango.

1 Preheat the oven to 200°C (180°C fan oven) mark 6. Grease a 33 × 23cm (13 × 9in) Swiss roll tin and line with baking parchment, then grease the paper. Dust with caster sugar and flour.
2 Put the eggs and sugar in a bowl, place over a pan of hot water and whisk with an electric hand whisk for 5 minutes until pale, creamy and thick enough to leave a trail on the surface when the whisk is lifted.
3 Remove the bowl from the heat and whisk until cool. Sift half the flour over the egg and sugar mixture and use a metal spoon to fold in lightly. Sift and fold in the remaining flour, then lightly stir in 1 tbsp hot water and the lime zest.
4 Pour the mixture into the tin and tilt it backwards and forwards to spread in an even layer. It may look very thin, but don't worry – it will rise. Bake in the oven for 10–12 minutes until golden, well risen and firm.
5 Meanwhile, put a large sheet of baking parchment on top of a damp tea towel and dredge the paper thickly with caster sugar. Quickly turn out the sponge on to the paper, then peel the baking parchment off the sponge. Trim the crusty edges, then leave to cool.
6 To make the filling, put the crème fraîche in a bowl, add the lime juice and mix. Spread over the sponge, then top with the mango slices.
7 Starting at a short edge, use the paper to roll up the sponge. Make the first turn firmly so it rolls evenly and has a good shape, but roll more lightly after this. Place seam-side down on a serving plate and dredge with sugar. Eat within a few hours.

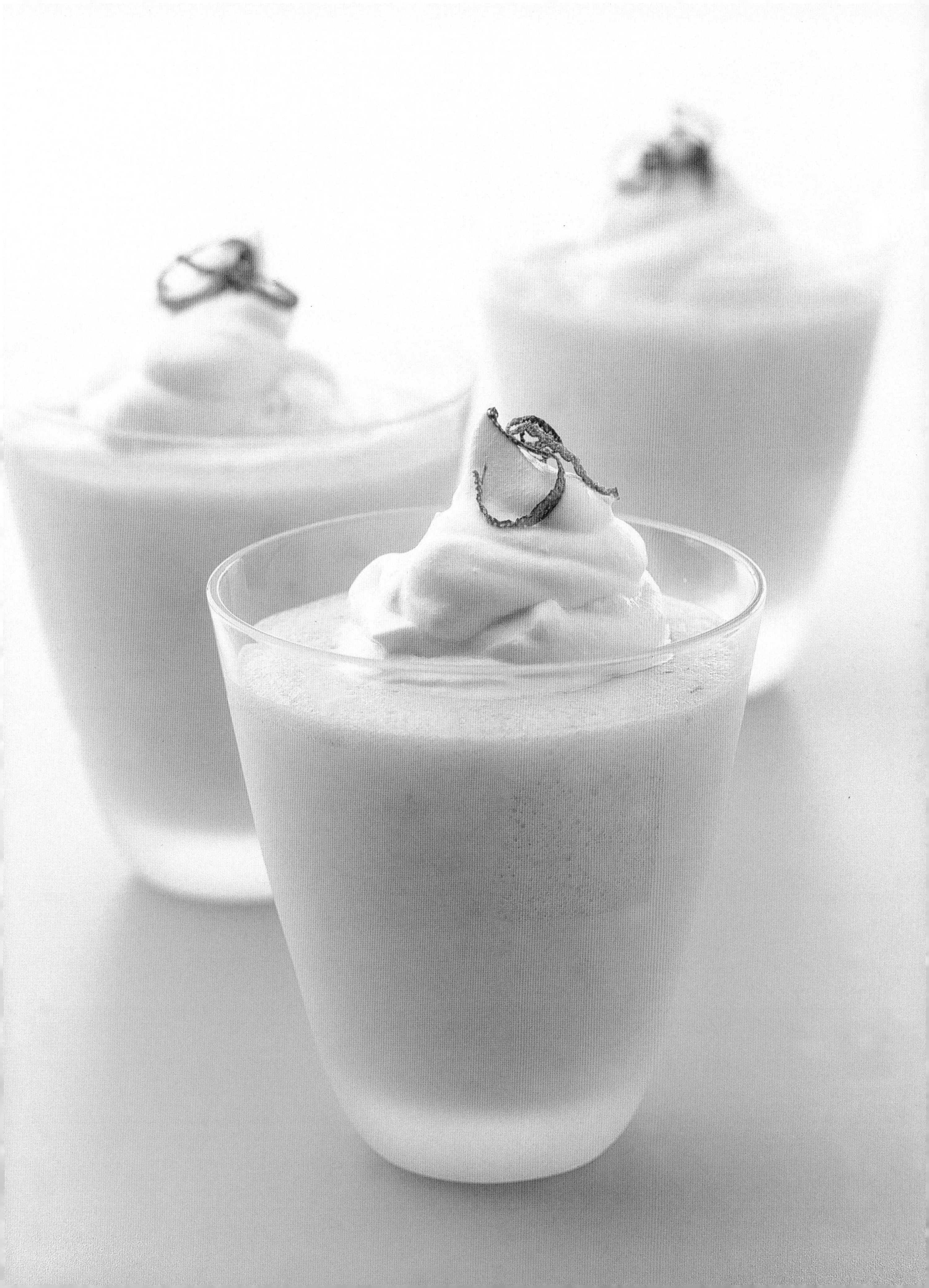

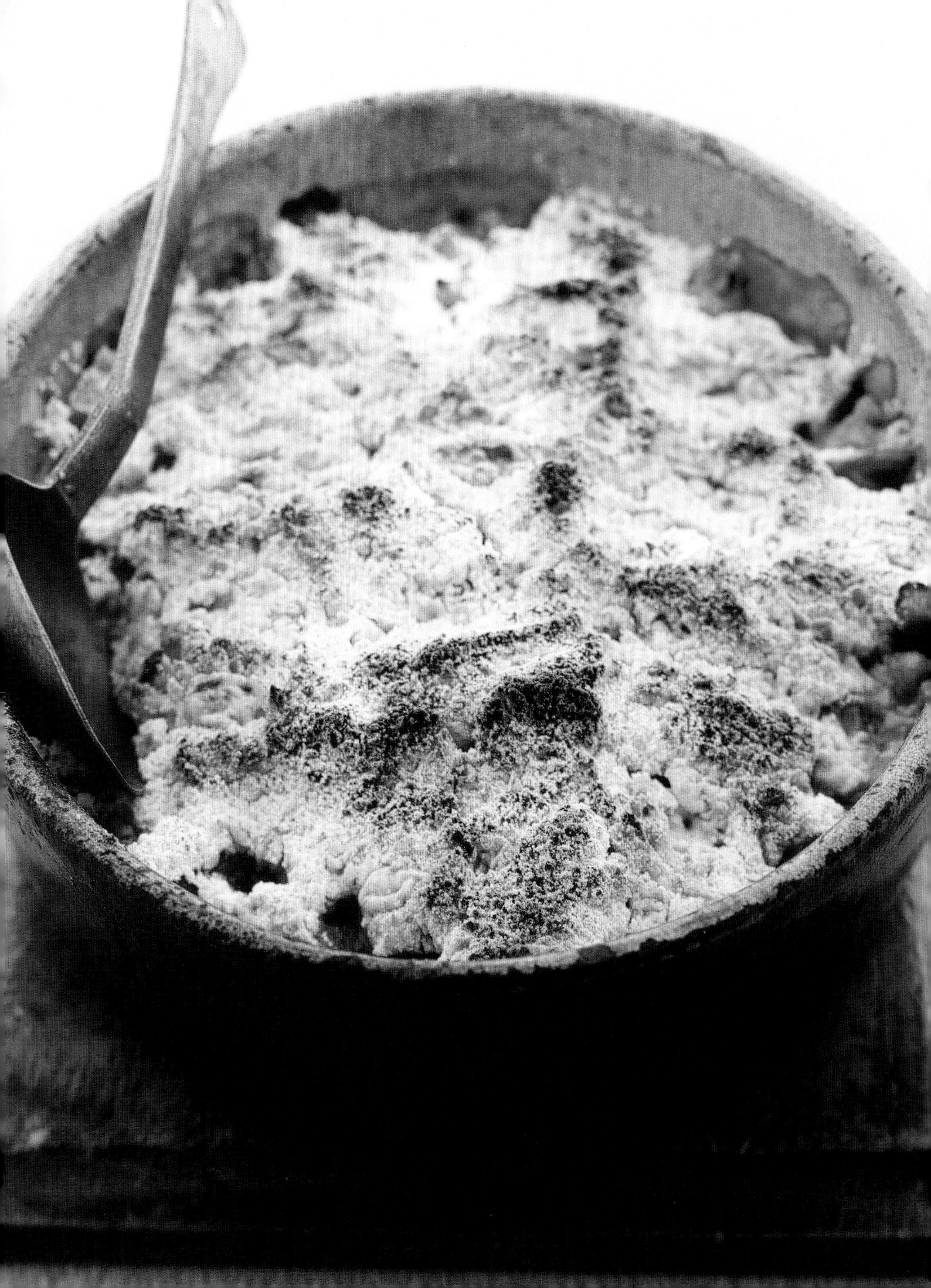

Rhubarb Crumble

450g (1lb) rhubarb, trimmed and chopped
2 balls stem ginger in syrup, drained and roughly chopped
125g (4½oz) light muscovado sugar
75g (3oz) reduced-fat spread
125g (4½oz) wholemeal flour

serves 8
preparation time: 15 minutes
cooking time: 45 minutes
per serving: 150 cals, 4g fat, 28g carbohydrate

Using light muscovado sugar in the topping gives the whole pudding a mellow, caramel flavour. The pieces of stem ginger add a refreshing bite to the rhubarb.

1 Preheat the oven to 180°C (160°C fan oven) mark 4. Put the rhubarb in a 1.1 litre (2 pint) pie dish. Mix in the stem ginger and sprinkle over half the sugar.
2 Put the reduced-fat spread and wholemeal flour in a food processor and whiz to make a coarse, breadcrumb-like mixture. Add the remaining sugar and pulse once or twice to mix together.
3 Spoon the topping over the fruit and bake for 50–60 minutes or until the pudding is golden brown and bubbling.

Spiced Pears in Mulled Wine Syrup

6 tbsp honey
4 tbsp light muscovado sugar
300ml (½ pint) full-bodied, fruity red wine
1 cinnamon stick or large pinch of ground cinnamon
Pared rind and juice of 1 large orange
6 small pears, ripe but firm

serves 6
preparation time: 20 minutes
cooking time: 15–20 minutes
per serving: 150 cals, 0g fat, 29g carbohydrate

TO FREEZE: Cool and freeze the cooked pears in the syrupy wine.
NOTE: Firm pears such as Comice and Conference are best for poaching. Try other spices in the syrup, such as sliced fresh root ginger or whole cloves.

Everyone loves the rich flavour and light texture of these boozy, festive pears – especially welcome after a meaty main course. The fruit can be cooked well ahead or frozen. Serve very simply with chilled crème fraîche or vanilla ice cream. Firm, slightly under-ripe pears offer a lower GI. Make sure you cook them until just soft but not mushy. Although this dish is served in a sugar syrup, note that if you eat it after a low GI high fibre meal, your blood glucose rise should still be slow and steady.

1 Mix together the honey, sugar, wine, cinnamon, orange rind and juice in a medium saucepan. Gently heat together until the sugar dissolves, bring to the boil, then reduce to a simmer.
2 Meanwhile, peel the pears with a vegetable peeler, leaving the stalks intact to make them easier to handle. Cut a thin slice from the base of each pear so that it sits upright. Lower into the wine.
3 Add enough water to just cover the pears and set a heatproof plate on top to keep them immersed in the liquid. Poach the pears at a gentle simmer for 20–25 minutes until tender when pierced with a knife.
4 Lift the cooked pears from the pan and lie flat in a serving dish. Put the saucepan back on the hob, bring to the boil and bubble for 15–20 minutes until the syrup has reduced and is syrupy. Strain the wine over the pears to colour them evenly, then cover with clingfilm and chill overnight (this allows the flavour and colour to intensify). Stand the pears upright in the syrup to serve.

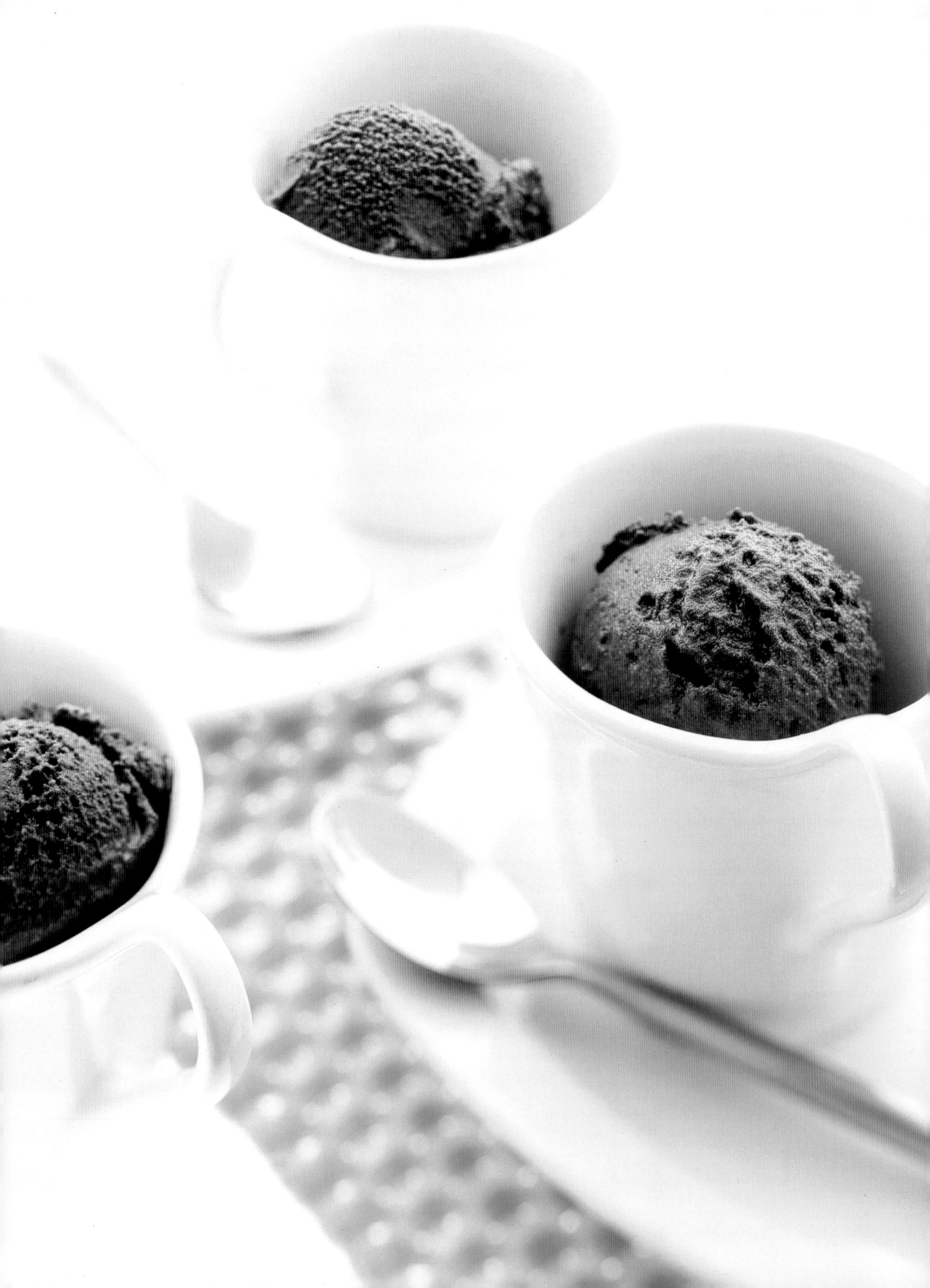

Chocolate Cinnamon Sorbet

200g (7oz) golden granulated sugar
50g (2oz) cocoa powder
Pinch of salt
1 tsp instant espresso coffee powder
1 cinnamon stick
6 tsp crème de cacao (chocolate liqueur) to serve

serves 8
preparation time: 5 minutes, plus chilling and freezing
cooking time: 15 minutes
per serving: 130 cals, 1g fat, 28g carbohydrate

This would make a great dessert to serve at a dinner party. Prepare beforehand to cut down on preparation on the day.

1 Put the sugar, cocoa powder, salt, coffee and cinnamon stick into a large pan with 600ml (1 pint) water. Bring to the boil, stirring until the sugar has completely dissolved. Boil for 5 minutes, then remove from the heat. Leave to cool. Remove the cinnamon stick, then chill.
2 If you have an ice-cream maker, put the mixture into it and churn for about 30 minutes until firm. Otherwise, pour into a freezerproof container and put in the coldest part of the freezer until firmly frozen, then transfer the frozen mixture to a blender or food processor and blend until smooth. Quickly put the mixture back in the container and return it to the freezer for at least 1 hour.
3 To serve, scoop the sorbet into individual cups and drizzle 1 tsp chocolate liqueur over each portion. Serve immediately.

Orange Sorbet

10 juicy oranges
200g (7oz) golden caster sugar
2 tbsp orange flower water
1 large egg white

serves 4–6
preparation time: 20 minutes, plus chilling and freezing
per serving: 300–200 cals, 0g fat, 76–51g carbohydrate

Refreshing and delicious.

1 Finely pare the zest from the oranges, using a citrus zester, then squeeze the juice. Put the zest and juice into a pan with the sugar and 200ml (7fl oz) water, and heat gently to dissolve the sugar. Increase the heat and boil for 1 minute. Set aside to cool.
2 Stir the orange flower water into the cooled sugar syrup. Cover and chill in the fridge for 30 minutes.
3 Strain the orange syrup into a bowl. In another bowl, beat the egg white until just frothy, then whisk into the orange mixture.
4 For best results, freeze in an ice-cream maker. Otherwise, pour into a shallow freezerproof container and freeze until almost frozen; mash well with a fork and freeze until solid. Transfer the sorbet to the fridge 30 minutes before serving to soften slightly.

Orange Meringue Terrine

meringue
5 large egg whites, at room temperature
275g (10oz) golden caster sugar
1 tsp orange juice
1 tsp cornflour, sifted
orange filling
2 tbsp cornflour, sifted
4 large egg yolks
100g (3¾oz) golden caster sugar
Finely grated zest and juice of 2 oranges
100ml (4fl oz) skimmed milk
150ml (¼ pint) whipping cream

serves 10-12
preparation time: 40 minutes
cooking time: 1 hour 35 minutes, plus cooling
per serving: 250-210 cals, 8-7g fat, 43-36g carbohydrate

Try this new alternative to the more traditional lemon meringue tart. Although it takes a long time to cook, it can be made a week ahead and frozen.

1 Draw three 25 × 10cm (10 × 4in) rectangles on baking parchment. Cut around the rectangles, leaving a 10cm (4in) border. Turn the paper over and put each rectangle on a baking sheet.
2 For the meringue, whisk the egg whites in a clean bowl until softly peaked. Whisk in the sugar, a tablespoonful at a time. Continue to beat until the meringue is glossy and firm. Fold in the orange juice and cornflour.
3 Put the meringue into a large piping bag fitted with a large star nozzle. Pipe widthways along each piece of parchment to create 3 oblongs. Pipe 4 stars on to another baking sheet lined with parchment.
4 Bake the meringue at 140°C (120°C fan oven) mark 1 for 20 minutes, then turn the oven down to 110°C (100°C fan oven) mark ¼ and bake for a further 1¼ hours. Turn the oven off and leave the meringue inside for 30 minutes to 1 hour to cool and dry out.
5 For the filling, mix the cornflour with 1 tbsp water in a bowl, then stir in the egg yolks, sugar, orange zest and juice. Bring the milk to the boil in a pan, then gradually stir into the cornflour mixture. Return it to the pan and cook, stirring constantly with a whisk, over a gentle heat, until it is very thick. Tip the custard into a bowl, cover the surface with wet greaseproof paper to prevent a skin forming, and allow to cool. Whip the cream until softly peaked, then fold into the custard.
6 Carefully lift the meringue shapes off the parchment. Use the orange custard to sandwich the 3 meringue layers together and place on a serving plate. Spoon 4 blobs of orange custard on the top layer and position the meringue stars on top. Cut into slices to serve.

Lemon Sorbet

3 juicy lemons
125g (4 oz) golden caster sugar
1 large egg white

serves 3–4
preparation time: 10 minutes, plus chilling and freezing
per serving: 170–130 cals, 0g fat, 45–34g carbohydrate

A favourite with many people, the fresh lemon flavour clears the taste buds at the end of a meal.

1 Finely pare the lemon zest, using a zester, then squeeze the juice. Put the zest in a pan with the sugar and 350ml (12fl oz) water and heat gently to dissolve. Increase the heat and boil for 10 minutes. Leave to cool.
2 Stir the lemon juice into the cooled sugar syrup. Cover and chill in the fridge for 30 minutes.
3 Strain the syrup through a fine sieve into a bowl. In another bowl, beat the egg white until it is just frothy, then whisk into the lemon mixture.
4 For best results, freeze in an ice-cream maker. Otherwise, pour into a shallow, freezer-proof container and freeze until almost frozen; mash well with a fork and freeze until solid. Transfer the sorbet to the fridge 30 minutes before serving to soften slightly.

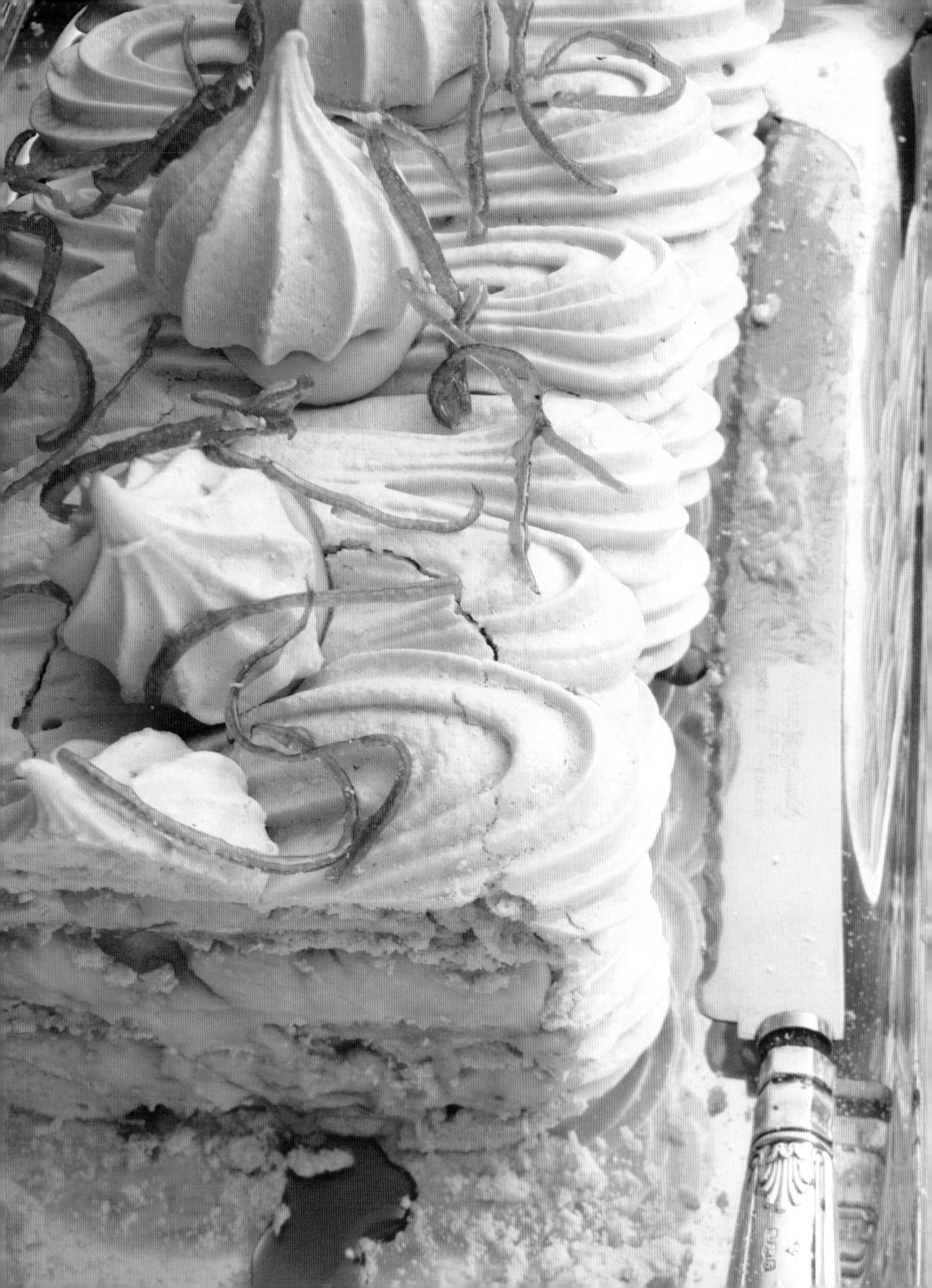

Fresh Vanilla Custard

600ml (1 pint) skimmed milk
1 vanilla pod or 1 tbsp vanilla extract
6 medium egg yolks
2 level tbsp golden caster sugar
2 tbsp cornflour

serves 8
preparation time: 10 minutes, plus 5 minutes' cooling time
cooking time: 10 minutes
per serving: 100 cals, 4g fat, 10g carbohydrate

As a special treat for the family, serve a real homemade custard – it tastes deliciously eggy.

1 Pour the milk into a pan. Cut a slit down the length of the vanilla pod and scrape the seeds into the pan with the pod, or pour in the vanilla extract. Bring to the boil. Turn off the heat immediately and leave to cool for 5 minutes.
2 Put the egg yolks, sugar and cornflour in a bowl and whisk together. Gradually whisk in the warm milk, leaving the vanilla pod behind if using.
3 Rinse the pan and pour the custard back in. Heat gently, whisking continuously for 2–3 minutes or until the mixture thickens – it should just coat the back of a wooden spoon in a thin layer. Serve immediately.

NOTE: If you want to prepare ahead, at the end of step 3, pour into a jug, cover the surface with a round of wet greaseproof paper, then cover with clingfilm and chill. To reheat, microwave in a 900W oven on MEDIUM for 2 minutes, stir, then microwave for 2 minutes.

Sparkling Fruit Jellies

75cl bottle demi-sec or dry sparkling wine
300ml (½ pint) red grape juice
5 tsp powdered gelatine
125g (4½oz) small seedless grapes, halved
225g (8oz) raspberries or small strawberries

serves 8
preparation time: 10 minutes, plus chilling time
per serving: 110 cals; trace fat; 10g carbohydrate

For a variation on this recipe, try using cranberry rather than grape juice.

1 Pour the sparkling wine into a bowl. Put 4 tbsp of the grape juice into a small pan, sprinkle the gelatine over it and leave to soak for 5 minutes, then heat very gently until the gelatine is completely dissolved. Stir in the remaining grape juice, then stir this mixture into the wine.
2 Divide the grapes and raspberries among serving glasses, pour in enough of the wine mixture to cover them and chill until just set.
3 Pour on the remaining wine mixture and chill for a further 3–4 hours until set.

Christmas Pudding Parfait

Finely grated zest and juice of 1 orange
2 tbsp brandy
125g (4oz) sultanas
125g (4oz) ready-to-eat prunes
1 tsp ground mixed spice
568ml carton whipping cream
4 large eggs, separated
125g (4oz) dark muscovado sugar, plus 1 tbsp extra
½ tsp vanilla extract

serves 14
preparation: 30 minutes, plus freezing
cooking time: 3–5 minutes
per serving: 340 cals; 25g fat; 26g carbohydrate

A great seasonal pudding and worthy alternative to the more traditional Christmas pudding.

1 Line a 2.3 litre (4 pint) pudding basin with clingfilm. Put the orange zest and juice, brandy, sultanas, prunes and mixed spice into a pan. Heat gently for 3–5 minutes until the liquid is absorbed and the fruit has plumped up. Tip into a food processor and whiz to a purée.
2 Whip the cream in a bowl until just thickened.
3 Whisk the egg yolks, 125g (4½oz) of the sugar and the vanilla extract together in another bowl, using an electric whisk, for 5 minutes until creamy and the sugar has dissolved. Using a metal spoon, fold in the whipped cream.
4 Whisk the egg whites in a clean bowl until soft peaks form. Beat in the 1 tbsp sugar. Stir a large spoonful into the egg and cream mixture, then fold in the rest with a metal spoon. Fold in the puréed fruit. Pour the mixture into the prepared pudding basin and freeze for 6 hours.
5 To serve, run the base of the bowl under a warm tap, turn out on to a serving plate and remove the clingfilm. Wrap the end of a holly sprig in clingfilm and insert into the parfait to decorate if you like.

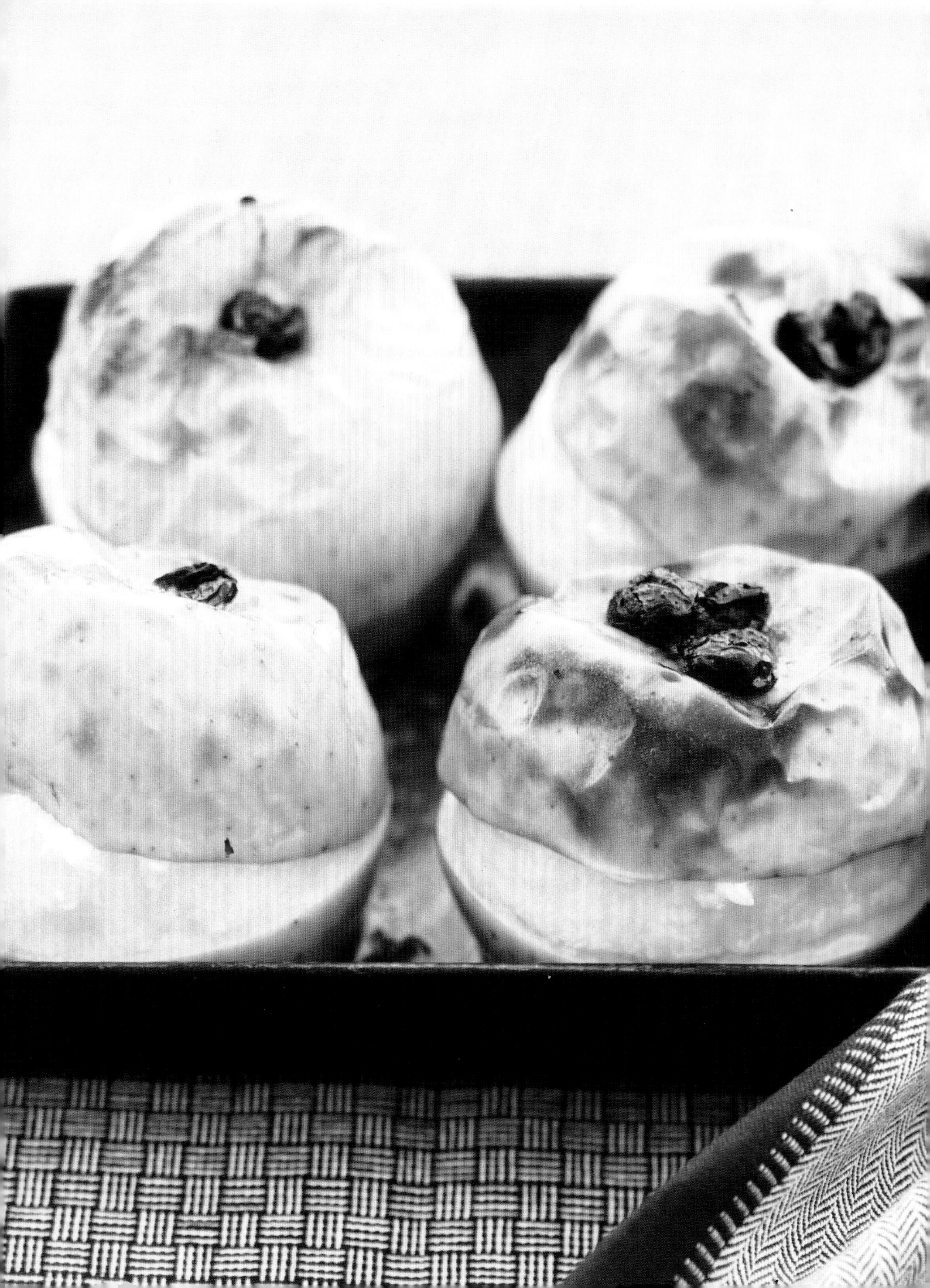

Baked Apples

4 small Bramley cooking apples
Zest and juice of 1 small orange
25g (1oz) light muscovado sugar
50g (2oz) dried cherries
25g (1oz) raisins
25g (1oz) butter

serves 4
preparation time: 10 minutes
cooking time: 30–35 minutes
per serving: 180 cals, 5g fat, 34g carbohydrate

Orange juice and dried cherries update this classic. Dollop a generous spoonful of low-fat Greek yogurt on top to serve.

1 Preheat the oven 200°C (180°C fan oven) mark 6. Core the apples, score them around the middle with a small, sharp knife (to prevent them exploding), then put them in a roasting pan or small ovenproof dish in which they fit quite snugly.
2 Stir together the orange zest and juice, muscovado sugar, dried cherries and raisins and divide into four, filling the space in each apple core.
3 Dot the apples with the butter and add 2tbsp water to the dish. Bake in the oven for 30–35 minutes or until they're soft. Transfer to serving plates, pour over the syrup from the dish and serve with low-fat Greek yogurt.

Grand Marnier Oranges and Passion Fruit

8 large, sweet oranges
6 passion fruit
100g (4½oz) golden caster sugar
4 tbsp Grand Marnier

serves 8
preparation time: 30 minutes
cooking time: 10 minutes
per serving: 120 cals, 0g fat, 26g carbohydrate

The great thing about this pudding is that the flavour is just as good if you make it two days in advance. Sharp, acidic fruit is the perfect antidote to a rich main course, and a glug of Grand Marnier adds a boozy touch to the syrup, while passion fruit give an exotic flavour. Serve with creamy crème fraîche.

1 Use a vegetable peeler to pare strips of peel from two oranges. Cut the strips into needle-fine shreds, then put into a heavy-based pan.
2 Cut the top and bottom off each orange, then use a sharp knife to remove all the skin and pith, and discard this. Slice the fruit into rounds, saving the juice, then put fruit into a bowl. Add the juice to the pan.
3 Cut each passion fruit in half. Scoop the juice and seeds of 3 fruits into the pan. Push the seeds and pulp of the remaining fruit through a sieve held over the pan, so the juice drips through; discard the seeds.
4 Add the caster sugar to the pan, set it over a medium heat and allow it to dissolve completely. Increase the heat and, swirling the pan occasionally, allow the sugar to caramelize gently – it should take about 10 minutes to become syrupy.
5 Remove the pan from the heat and add the Grand Marnier to the syrup – it may splutter as you do this, so protect your hands with a cloth. Cool the syrup, then pour it over the oranges. Cover and chill for up to two days before serving.

Passion Fruit and Strawberry Terrine

225g (8oz) ripe strawberries
5 large oranges
5 pink grapefruit
8 passion fruit
2 tbsp powdered gelatine
150g (5oz) golden caster sugar
to finish
Strawberries
Mint leaves

serves 8
preparation time: 50 minutes, plus chilling
cooking time: 2–3 minutes
per serving: 140 cals, 0g fat, 34g carbohydrate

Try this tasty combination of oranges, grapefruit, passion fruit and strawberries in an unusual dessert.

1 Halve the strawberries (or quarter if large). Squeeze the juice from 3 of the oranges. Using a sharp knife, cut the peel and pith from the grapefruit and remaining oranges, then cut into segments. Squeeze the juice from the membranes and add to the orange juice. Put the segments in a colander on a plate to catch the juice and leave to stand for 30 minutes. Halve the passion fruit and scoop out the pulp.
2 Pour 5 tbsp cold water into a small, heatproof bowl, sprinkle on the gelatine and set aside to soak for 5 minutes.
3 Put the passion fruit pulp and 2 tbsp of the orange juice in a food processor and pulse for 1 minute. Strain into a measuring jug and make up to 600ml (1 pint) with the remaining juice. Pour into a pan, then add the sugar. Heat gently to dissolve, then bring to the boil. Remove from the heat, add the soaked gelatine and stir until dissolved.
4 Line a 1.4 litre (2½ pint) terrine or loaf tin with clingfilm. Mix the grapefruit and orange segments together with the strawberries and spoon into the mould. Strain enough warm juice mixture over it to cover the fruit completely, then gently tap the mould to expel any air bubbles. Cover with clingfilm and chill for at least 6 hours, preferably overnight, until set.
5 To serve, turn the terrine out on to a board and cut into slices with a hot, serrated knife. Decorate with strawberries and mint.

Moist Carrot Cake

250ml (8fl oz) sunflower oil, plus extra to oil
225g (8oz) light muscovado sugar
3 large eggs
225g (8oz) self-raising flour
Large pinch of salt
½ tsp ground mixed spice
½ tsp ground nutmeg
½ tsp ground cinnamon
250g (9oz) carrots, peeled and coarsely grated

makes 12 slices
preparation time: 15 minutes
cooking time: 50–60 minutes, plus cooling
per slice: 330 cals, 20g fat, 35g carbohydrate

This version of the classic carrot cake has been adapted to work for a diabetic diet and is eaten without the rich icing.

1 Oil and base-line a 20cm (8in) round cake tin with greaseproof paper. Lightly oil the paper.
2 Using a hand-held electric whisk, whisk the oil and muscovado sugar together to combine, then whisk in the eggs, one at a time.
3 Sift the flour, salt and spices together over the mixture, then gently fold in, using a large metal spoon. Tip the grated carrot into the bowl and fold in.
4 Divide the cake mixture between the prepared tins and bake at 180°C (160°C fan oven) mark 4 for 50–60 minutes or until golden and a skewer inserted into the centre comes out clean. Leave in the tin for 10 minutes, then turn out on to a wire rack to cool.

NOTE: The cake will keep for up to a week in an airtight tin.

Strawberry Sorbet

250g (9oz) golden caster sugar
450g (1lb) sweet ripe strawberries
1 tbsp balsamic vinegar
1 large egg white

serves 4–6
preparation time: 20 minutes, plus chilling and freezing
per serving: 280–190 cals, 0g fat, 73–48g carbohydrate

1 Put the sugar and 250ml (9fl oz) water in a pan and heat gently to dissolve the sugar. Increase the heat and boil for 1 minute. Cool, then chill for 30 minutes.
2 Meanwhile, purée the strawberries in a blender or food processor, then pass through a sieve to remove the seeds. Cover and chill for 30 minutes.
3 Stir the sugar syrup and balsamic vinegar into the strawberry purée.
4 In another bowl, beat the egg white until just frothy, then whisk into the strawberry mixture.
5 For best results, freeze in an ice-cream maker. Otherwise, pour into a shallow freezerproof container and freeze until almost frozen; mash well with a fork and freeze until solid. Transfer the sorbet to the fridge 30 minutes before serving to soften slightly.

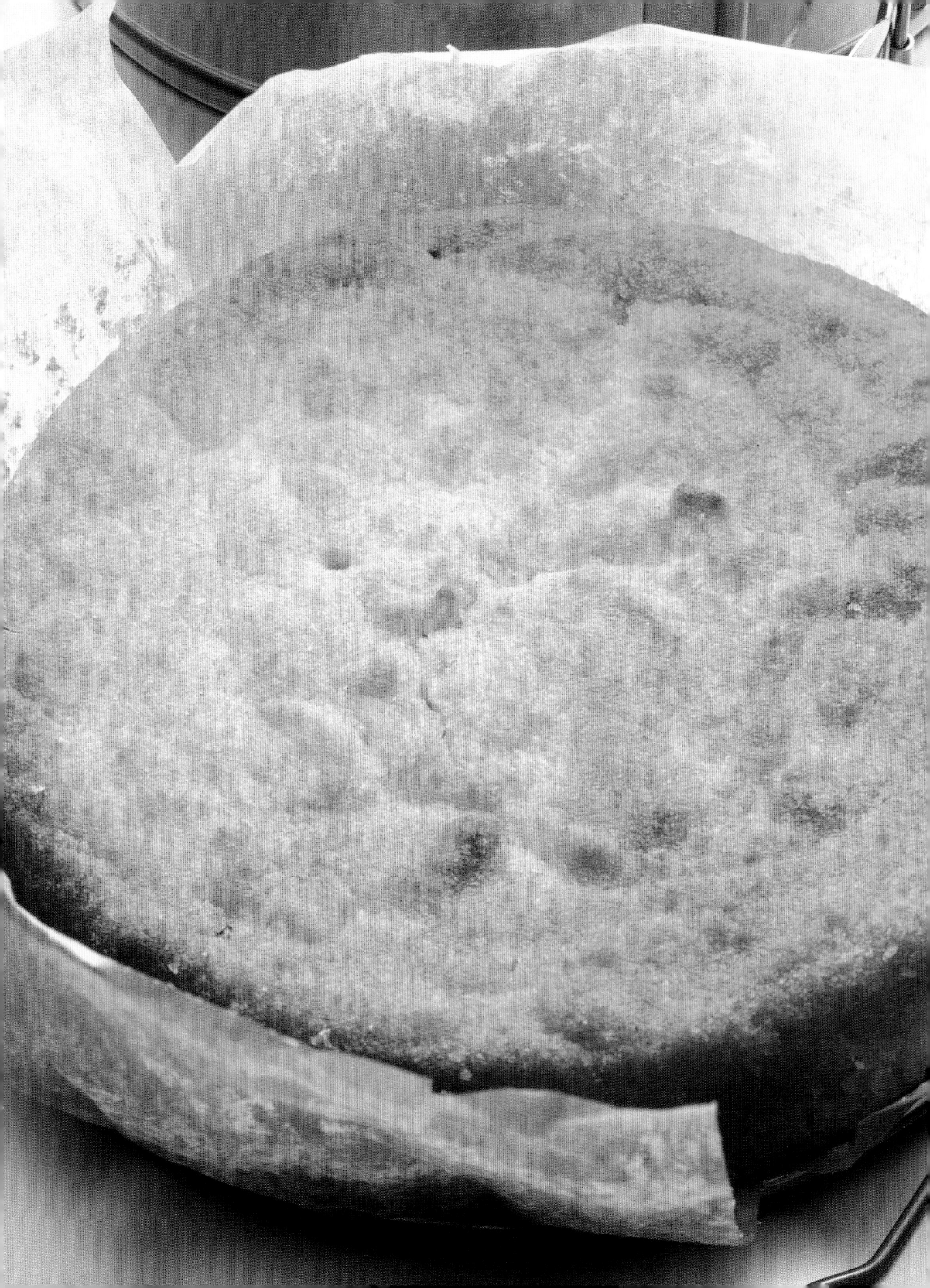

Almond and Orange Torte

Vegetable oil, to oil
Flour, to dust
1 medium orange
3 medium eggs
225g (8oz) golden caster sugar
250g (9oz) ground almonds
½ tsp baking powder
Icing sugar, to dust

makes 10 slices
preparation: 30 minutes
cooking time: 1 hour 50 minutes, plus cooling
per slice: 265 cals; 16g fat, 25g carbohydrate

A whole orange, boiled and then puréed, is the secret ingredient in this moist, tangy cake.

1 Grease and line, then oil and flour a 20cm (8in) spring-release cake tin.
2 Put the whole orange into a small pan and cover with water. Bring to the boil. Cover and simmer for at least 1 hour until tender. Drain and cool.
3 Cut the orange in half and remove the pips. Whiz in a food processor to make a smooth purée.
4 Put the eggs and sugar into a bowl and whisk together until thick and pale. Fold in the ground almonds, baking powder and orange purée.
5 Pour the mixture into the prepared tin. Bake at 180°C (160°C fan oven) mark 4 for 40–50 minutes or until a skewer inserted into the centre comes out clean. Leave to cool in the tin.
6 Unclip the tin and remove the lining paper from the cake. Dust with icing sugar and serve cut into slices. It can be served with low-fat Greek yogurt.

Rice Pudding

butter, to grease
125g (4oz) short-grain pudding rice
1.2 litres (2 pints) semi skimmed milk
50g (2oz) golden caster sugar
Grated zest of 1 orange (optional)
1 tsp vanilla extract
Freshly grated nutmeg, to taste

serves 6
preparation: 5 minutes
cooking time: 1½ hours
per serving: 200 cals; 3g fat; 35g carbohydrate

A delicious and warming traditional pudding.

1 Lightly butter a 1.5 litre (2¾ pint) ovenproof dish. Add the pudding rice, milk, sugar, orange zest if using, and vanilla extract and stir everything together. Grate the nutmeg over the top of the mixture.
2 Bake the pudding in the middle of the oven at 170°C (150°C fan oven) mark 3 for 1½ hours or until the top is golden brown.

NOTE: Orange zest gives the pudding a fruity tang, but you can leave it out for a more traditional flavour.

Blueberry muffins

300g (11oz) plain flour
2 level teaspoons baking powder
150g (5oz) golden caster sugar
finely grated zest of 1 lemon
125g (4oz) dried blueberries
1 medium egg
1 teaspoon vanilla extract
225ml (8fl oz) skimmed milk
50g (2Oz) unsalted butter

makes 10
preparation: 15 minutes
cooking time: 20–25 minutes, plus cooling
250 cals, 6g fat, 50g carbohydrate

Using dried blueberries instead of fresh in this recipe will mean that less juice is released and stop your muffins turning grey inside.

1 Line a muffin tin with 10 paper muffin cases.
2 Sift the flour and baking powder together into a bowl. Stir in the caster sugar, lemon zest and dried blueberries.
3 Put the egg, vanilla extract, milk and melted butter into a jug and mix together with a fork. Pour this liquid into the dry ingredients and lightly fold together – don't overmix.
4 Spoon the mixture into the muffin cases to three-quarters fill them. Bake at 200°C (180°C fan) mark 6 for 20–25 minutes until the muffins are risen, pale golden and just firm.
5 Transfer to a wire rack and leave to cool slightly. Dust with icing sugar to serve.

Fruity Rice Pudding

125g (4oz) pudding rice
1.1 litres (2 pints) skimmed milk
1 teaspoon vanilla extract
3–4 level tablespoons caster sugar
200ml (7fl oz) ricotta cheese
12 level tablespoons wild lingonberry sauce

makes 12
preparation: 10 minutes, plus 30 minutes cooling and minimum 1 hour chilling
cooking time: 1 hour
390 cals, 20g fat, 46g carbohydrate

The sharp lingonberry sauce contrasts wonderfully with the creamy rice in this pudding.

1 Put the rice in a pan with 600ml (1 pint) cold water, bring to the boil and simmer until the liquid has evaporated. Add the milk, bring to the boil and simmer for 45 minutes or until the rice is very soft and creamy. Cool.
2 Add the vanilla extract and sugar to the rice. Lightly whip the ricotta cheese and fold through the pudding. Chill for 1 hour.
3 Divide a third of the rice mixture between six tumblers, top with a spoonful of lingonberry sauce and repeat the process, finishing with the rice. Chill until ready to serve.

Instant Banana Ice Cream

6 bananas, about 700g (1½lb), peeled, cut into thin slices and frozen
1–2 tablespoons virtually fat-free fromage frais
1–2 tablespoons orange juice
1 teaspoon natural vanilla extract
Splash of rum or Cointreau (optional)
A few drops of lime juice to taste

makes 4
preparation: 5 minutes plus freezing
176 cals

Frozen banana makes the creamiest instant ice cream you can imagine – it tastes indulgent but is low in fat.

1 Leave the frozen banana to stand at room temperature for 2–3 minutes. Put the still frozen pieces in a food processor with 1 tablespoon fromage frais, 1 tablespoon orange juice, vanilla extract and the liqueur.
2 Whiz until smooth, scraping down the sides of the bowl and adding more fromage frais and orange juice as necessary to give a creamy consistency.
3 Serve at once or turn into a freezer container and freeze for up to one month.

To freeze bananas
Peel and slice thinly, then put the banana on a large non-stick baking tray and place in the freezer for 30 minutes or until frozen. Transfer to a plastic bag and store in a freezer until needed.

Further information and support

Books

Think Well To Be Well, Azmina Govindji and Nina Puddefoot (Diabetes Research & Wellness Foundation, 2002).

The GI Plan, lose weight forever, Azmina Govindji and Nina Puddefoot (Vermilion, 2004).

Other *Good Housekeeping* titles

30-Minute Suppers
(Collins & Brown, 2005)

Preserves (Collins & Brown, 2005)

Cookery Book (Collins & Brown, 2004)

One-Pot Cooking
(Collins & Brown, 2003)

Short Cuts for Busy Cooks
(Collins & Brown, 2003)

Websites

www.giplan.com

This is a supportive site for anyone wanting to get into GI eating by using the GI Plan and motivational strategies.

www.thinkwelltobewell.com

This website offers golden nuggets of information and inspires you to check and challenge your thinking, it offers willpower boosters, slimming tips, and a host of information on diet and diabetes.

The British Dietetic Association sites include:

www.bda.uk.com
www.weightwisebda.uk.com

For diabetes-specific sites, visit:

www.diabeteswellnessnet.org.uk
www.diabetes.org.uk

Contacts

Registered dietitians hold the only legally recognisable graduate qualification in nutrition and dietetics. If you would like to visit a dietitian, ask your GP to refer you or contact:

British Dietetic Association
5th Floor, Charles House
148/9 Great Charles Street
Queensway
Birmingham B3 3HT
Tel: 0121 200 8080

Diabetes Research and Wellness Foundation (DRWF)
The DRWF is a charity working to relieve the suffering of people with diabetes and related illnesses.

Diabetes Research and Wellness Foundation
Northney Marina
Hayling Island
Hants
PO11 ONH
Tel: 023 9263 7808

Diabetes and food index

Recipe index

Photographers

Marie Louise Avery pages 17, 42, 107; Steve Baxter pages 9, 13, 14, 22, 31, 54, 58, 60, 82, 94, 122, 124, 130; John Blythe page 67; Jean Cazals page 70; Sian Irvine page 52; David Jones page 56; William Lingwood page 121; Jonathan Lovekin pages 40, 73; David Munns pages 28, 33; Michael Paul pages 6, 80, 84, 111; Lucinda Symons page 49; Martin Thompson pages 37, 38, 64, 77, 105, 109, 118, 127, 134; Elizabeth Zeschin page 103

Acknowledgements

Several people have helped me to create this resource and to reach a level of expertise that enables me to apply my knowledge appropriately. Firstly, I must acknowledge my previous manager and role model from way back in the late 80s, Lynne Graham. I then worked as a diabetes dietitian in Ealing Health Authority and it was Lynne who had the confidence in me and pushed me to apply for the Chief Dietitian position at Diabetes UK. I would also like to thank my colleagues, Sue Baic and Rebecca Chandler, who have skilfully helped with some parts of the introduction. Thanks to James Rogers of the Diabetes Research and Wellness Foundation for constantly being willing to support me and collaborate with me on my diabetes-related projects. Credit also goes to Nicola Hodgson of Chrysalis Books, who has shown tolerance and co-operation during the stressful periods leading up to publication. Most of all, I am grateful to my husband, Shamil, who has always been there to encourage me.